MW00466652

Cannabis and the Ch[r]
ful, biblical, and enjo[y]
with the conclusions,
to think through how ..
of our day, and Todd Miles has given us a helpful tool.

Sean McDowell, PhD, Biola University
professor, speaker, and author

The question of what to do about legalized marijuana has reached the church's doorstep. Todd Miles provides a skilled and timely answer. He is fiercely biblical in his treatment, clear in his warnings, and tender with those looking for relief in the midst of suffering. But he does so much more than address cannabis use. Miles models how to think Christianly about ethics when the Bible doesn't offer a proof text, how to lean into God and his Word when we experience chronic pain, and how to react when the demands of the government don't align with the demands of God. Pick up this book as soon as you can! If the problems Miles addresses aren't knocking on the door of your church and family right now, they will be very soon.

Aaron Menikoff, PhD, senior pastor, Mount Vernon
Baptist Church, Atlanta, Georgia, and author of *Character
Matters: Shepherding in the Fruit of the Spirit*

More than ever before, it is critically important to be a thinking Christian. It's so easy for our responses to questions to be based on opinions or emotions, or to not think about it too much and go with whatever the strongest voices are—even if they're not biblically thoughtful or well researched. What I love about Todd's book is that it is extremely thoughtful. Foremost, it is biblically based, but it really looks at the reality of marijuana usage today, not in a shallow or reactionary way, but in the context of scientific and cultural insight. I'm thankful to finally have a book I can now recommend and use in day-to-day life and ministry on this topic.

Dan Kimball, author of *How (Not) to Study
the Bible* and Western Seminary faculty

We are called to take every thought and action captive to Christ. Therefore, as states continue to legalize marijuana, the question becomes, *How are we to think biblically about Mary Jane?* Though the Bible doesn't address it directly, Miles argues the Bible is sufficient to address the issue. The research on marijuana is a moving target, but Miles provides a wise and winsome Christian analysis of both recreational and medical marijuana. Discipleship must include dealing with tough current issues, and Miles is a shepherd along the path. Pick up a few copies of this book and pass it around to parents, teens, and pastors.

Patrick Schreiner, PhD, associate professor of New Testament and Biblical Theology, Midwestern Baptist Theological Seminary and author of *The Visual Word: Illustrated Outlines of the New Testament Books*

With the de-stigmatization and often recreational legalization of marijuana sweeping across the American landscape, it is easy to treat significant issues as old hat and simply as part of the "new consensus." Todd Miles's book is a welcome rebuttal to what will likely be an issue that will have tremendous impact on the local church and throughout American culture. He does a fine job of exploring the overt and implicit dangers linked with marijuana use and does so by appealing to scriptural authority.

Andrew T. Walker, PhD, associate professor of Christian Ethics, The Southern Baptist Theological Seminary

Todd Miles has done the Christian and the local pastor an enormous service with this book. With clarity, precision, and pastoral sensitivity, he addresses the legal, medical, moral, and ethical questions facing Christians in a culture hurtling toward widespread legalization of marijuana. This book distills and presents the careful, nuanced wisdom of Scripture to help followers of Jesus answer the questions posed by legalization. But more than that, Todd calls us to a faithful discipleship which understands the relief of suffering is not our highest goal, but rather joy in the Lord. I highly recommend this book.

Michael Lawrence, lead pastor of Hinson Baptist Church, Portland, Oregon

CANNABIS

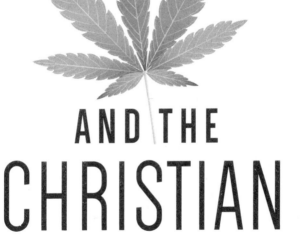

AND THE

CHRISTIAN

CANNABIS

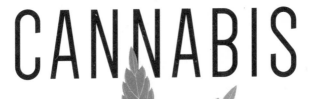

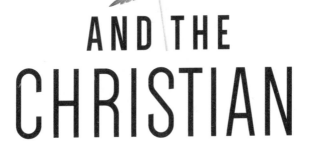

AND THE
CHRISTIAN

What the Bible Says about Marijuana

TODD MILES

B&H
PUBLISHING
NASHVILLE, TENNESSEE

978-1-0877-3496-5

Published by B&H Publishing Group
Nashville, Tennessee

Dewey Decimal Classification: 633.7
Subject Heading: MARIJUANA / MEDICAL ETHICS /
RECREATION

Design by B&H Publishing Group.
Illustration by okamigo/123rf.

1 2 3 4 5 6 • 25 24 23 22 21

Acknowledgments

The people at B&H have been kind to me the past few years. They cared for me and my family when my wife was ill and have been a source of encouragement to me in my writing. I'm grateful for Taylor Combs who believed in the timeliness of this project and has worked hard to turn my writing into a useful book. Thanks also to Devin Maddox, Stacey Sapp, and all those behind the scenes who have worked hard to make this book the best it can be.

I had a great team of people who read all of my chapter drafts and commented on them. That team included Tracy Fabel, Taylor Turkington, Kelli Templeton, Josh and Dizzie Hus, Lee Watkins, Anthony and Natalie Locke, Trent Hughes, Christian Lawrence, and Ron Marrs. *Cannabis and the Christian* is clearer and more pastoral because of them.

My oldest sons were especially helpful. Ethan was my "science and medicine" editor who made sure my explanations were both understandable and accurate. Levi read all my initial chapter drafts and cleaned them up for me.

Finally, a special thank you must go to my wife, Camille. She encouraged me to write and then created the space for me to do so, all while in the middle of chemotherapy and radiation therapy. She even gave me permission to reference her struggles in the chapter on suffering. Camille has always been my toughest and, therefore, best first reader. This book is no exception. I am exceedingly grateful to her and for her.

Contents

Introduction | 1

Chapter 1 | 15
What Is Marijuana and How Does It Work?

Chapter 2 | 30
The Risks of Marijuana Use

Chapter 3 | 52
The Christian and the Law

Chapter 4 | 69
The Bible and Marijuana

Chapter 5 | 90
Discipleship and Marijuana

Chapter 6 | 115
How Does Medical Marijuana Work?

Chapter 7 | 129
Thinking Biblically about Medical Marijuana

Appendix | 154
Questions and Answers for Pastors and Parents

Introduction

In December 2012, recreational marijuana was legalized in the state of Washington, a short drive across the mighty Columbia River from my neighborhood in Portland, Oregon. That week a member of the church where I was serving as an elder contacted the leaders to ask if it would be permissible, now that marijuana was legal, for him to drive across the bridge to smoke some pot.

If this question had been asked just a month or so earlier, the answer would have been obvious: "No, it's against the law." But now violation of the law could no longer be given as the reason for abstaining.[1] So, what were we to say? Churches could no longer bind the consciences of Christians to abstain from marijuana by appealing to

---

[1] Marijuana is currently listed as a Schedule 1 drug by the federal government, making the possession and/or selling of marijuana a violation of federal law. But the federal government is on record as refusing to enforce the federal marijuana ban against individuals who comply with state laws.

governmental prohibitions. A more thoughtful response would be required.

A few months later I was asked to do a breakout session at a pastor's conference, where I had spoken annually on theological and ethical hot topics—contemporary issues pastoral leaders had to confront. I decided to address the issue of the church and marijuana.

In the opening program the breakout leaders were asked to give a little advertisement for their sessions. When I announced that I was going to be speaking on the topic of "Marijuana and the Minister," the assembly erupted in laughter. Throughout the next day, before my breakout session, I was given title recommendations: "The Deacon and the Doobie," "The Trinity and Tree," "The Pastor and Pot," "Weed and the Way," "The Bible and the Blunt," "The Gospel and Grass." I could go on and on. Many of the recommendations were funny, but I did wonder if anybody was going to take the topic seriously and show up.

They did.

My breakout session was packed, every chair taken, with people overflowing into the hallway.

Since then, in addition to speaking about the topic on podcasts and radio shows, I have delivered the "Cannabis and the Christian" talk to churches, men's groups, youth groups, and conferences in Washington, Oregon,

Montana, and California. Initially, I just addressed recreational marijuana. Later, I added a separate talk on medical marijuana. Without exception, every time I speak on the topic, the Q&A at the end runs later than the time allotted. This issue is clearly on the minds of followers of Jesus around the country.

The Church Has Some Catching Up to Do

Churches have ignored the issue of marijuana for far too long. The reason, I believe, is threefold.

First, to many in the church, it was just self-evident that marijuana use was sinful, and the question was not even worth considering. If people did have questions, they were ashamed or embarrassed to ask. Dismissal might have been possible in the past, but our current context demands that the question now be considered.

Second, because marijuana possession and distribution were illegal at both the federal and state level for so long, churches did not have to think theologically about marijuana; they could simply appeal to those laws that prohibited marijuana use when counseling or discipling church members. As those state prohibitions have begun to disappear, so has the default argument of many churches.

Third, the Bible does not specifically address marijuana, either positively or negatively. Because Scripture neither explicitly promotes nor forbids the use of marijuana, it requires heavier lifting to present theological arguments. When you can't quote chapter and verse, it's more challenging to glean biblical wisdom on a topic.

> **Because marijuana possession and distribution were illegal at both the federal and state level for so long, churches did not have to think theologically about marijuana.**

But If Marijuana Is Not in the Bible . . .

All of this raises a good question: If the Bible does not explicitly mention marijuana or any other name for the cannabis or hemp plant, how can one write a book subtitled *What the Bible Says about Marijuana* and have something other than a book full of blank pages?

The answer: very carefully.

Let me explain.

I understand that the Bible is the Word of the living God. It is inspired by God and is therefore without errors. Further, I believe the Bible is sufficient. By that I mean that God has given to us all the divine words we need to live faithfully before him, even today. Notice that I did not say that we have all the divine words we might want. There are plenty of areas where I would love a few more divine words. For example, the creation of the cosmos is basically covered on one page of my Bible. I would love to have more revelation of what happened and how. But God, in his infinite wisdom, has deemed what Genesis 1 communicates to be sufficient for us to live faithfully before him.

Initially, we might think it would be nice to have a word from God that exactly matches the specific needs of the moment. But think about it: Do you want cookbook instructions for every possible circumstance? Imagine how long such Bibles would have to be! On reflection, we ought to agree that God's wisdom ought not to be called into question, as he has instead laid a foundation of divine revelation from which growth in godliness and wisdom can be achieved. Due to the historical and cultural context in which the Scriptures were written, marijuana is not specifically mentioned, but the Bible has much to say about things like discipleship, wisdom, mind-altering substances, human needs, human frailty, stewardship, creation, and addiction. What the Bible says on these topics will provide wisdom on the question of marijuana.

God has given us all the divine words we need to faithfully navigate the issues surrounding marijuana and the church. In the following pages, I want to use correct biblical interpretation to specifically answer the questions surrounding both recreational and medical marijuana. In

God has given us all the divine words we need to faithfully navigate the issues surrounding marijuana and the church.

so doing, I also hope to model a more general skill: how to think biblically about something that is not specifically in the Bible.

This Book Is (Primarily) for Christians

A quick word is in order regarding whom this book is for. It is primarily for Christians. Many of my arguments and considerations will be applicable to all people, regardless of whether they understand themselves to be Christians. After all, the medical risks for unbelievers are the same as those for believers. But most of my arguments are aimed at Christians.

A Christian is a follower of Jesus.

You are probably thinking that the previous sentence is obvious, but this assertion is vital to grasp before we move forward. Acts 11:26 teaches that the name "Christian" was first used of the disciples of Jesus in Antioch during the first century. By the time we get to Acts 11, the epicenter of Christian missions had moved from Jerusalem up to Antioch, and this church was responsible for sending out the apostle Paul on his first missionary journey. That church was committed to following Christ, and those disciples (or "learners") of Christ were called Christians. So a Christian is a disciple, a learner, a follower of Jesus.

The one the Christian follows, Jesus, is none other than the second member of the Trinity, God in the flesh. He is described as the "King of Kings and Lord of Lords" (Rev. 19:16), so the Christian view of Jesus is pretty high. One becomes a Christian by confessing that Jesus is Lord and believing that God raised him from the dead (Rom. 10:9).

Jesus is not just a wise man walking around dropping wisdom that can be considered and either accepted or rejected. He has authority, and he demands that his followers listen and obey. Jesus is Lord.

But Jesus is also good. The Bible teaches that Jesus is compassionate (Mark 6:34), gentle (Matt. 21:5), and loving (John 11:1–5). Jesus describes himself as the good shepherd, the one who lays down his life for his sheep (John 10:11). And of course, that is exactly what he did. Jesus died for our sins and rose again to save us. It was an act of self-sacrificing, humiliating, and gloriously wonderful love. Here is no omnipotent yet brutal, authoritarian taskmaster, ruthlessly commanding those weaker than him to do his selfish bidding. Jesus is all-powerful, but he is simultaneously meek and mild.

Here is how his disciple and friend Matthew described him, using the prediction of the prophet Isaiah. "He will not argue or shout, and no one will hear his voice in the streets. He will not break a bruised reed, and he will not put out a smoldering wick, until he has led justice to victory. The nations will put their hope in his name" (Matt. 12:19–21).

Further, Jesus Christ is wise. How wise? Paul described Jesus this way: "In him are hidden all the treasures of wisdom and knowledge" (Col. 2:3). Bottom line: Jesus is worth your trust.

Jesus demonstrated his love for his people by dying for them, and he continually demonstrates that love through his care, provision, and guidance. In response, Christians best demonstrate their love for Jesus, according to Jesus himself, by obeying him (John 14:21). All that to say, obedience to the words of Christ, either from his own lips or by his prophets and apostles, is crucial to the Christian life.

> The Christian should be deeply concerned about what Jesus thinks about marijuana. The difficulty lies in discerning what those thoughts might be.

So the Christian should be deeply concerned about what Jesus thinks about marijuana. The difficulty lies in discerning what those thoughts might be. That is the task of this book.

This Book and You

Before we begin, I want to offer a word of caution. Be aware that as you read I may say things either stronger than or not as strong as you might like. Some will be disappointed in my conclusions, believing them to allow too much. Others will be shocked at how restrictive I am. Please recognize that you do not come to this issue as a blank slate, waiting for information so you can form a position for the first time. You already have thoughts and opinions on marijuana, and those form a position that you all hold with varying degrees of certainty. You hold your current position on marijuana because of what you have heard, what you have seen, and what you have experienced. This book is one more contribution, and I pray that it will be helpful to you.

Some of you will read this, already convinced that marijuana is evil, looking for more ammunition to share with your friends or children. Some of you believe marijuana is of great benefit. Perhaps you or someone you know was helped by medical marijuana. Maybe you believe you function best when smoking pot. Some of you might believe that using marijuana has deepened your spiritual life. Whatever your ideas coming into the reading of this book, recognize they will shape how you receive what you are about to read.

I remember doing a seminar at a normal gospel-preaching church one evening and staying behind to answer more questions than could be addressed in the allotted Q&A time. Two lines quickly formed, both equally angry for opposite reasons. One line contained people frustrated that I was so negative about marijuana. The other line was full of those equally frustrated that I was so accommodating of marijuana. Both sets of people heard the same presentation but heard it in two different ways. As the people presented their cases, their pastor would often interject, "But Todd did not say that!" They were confident they heard what I did not say.

There is a lot of misinformation and confusion about marijuana. Many who read this will be surprised to hear of the risks associated with marijuana consumption. I have been careful to cite credible medical and legal sources for the claims I have made. You can find them in the footnotes.

Our experiences shape our convictions, and they color the way we see and hear things. So I invite you to read this book with your Bible open in front of you. Evaluate how I am interpreting the Scriptures to see if my conclusions and recommendations are faithful.

I am convinced the people of God need more Bible teaching, not less. We need to teach with a loud voice all the things the Scriptures clearly teach. But we also need to teach with a softer voice where the Bible is less clear. Pastors and teachers have been given the right and responsibility to bind the consciences of the people of God to obey him where he has spoken. But we must be careful not to abuse that responsibility in areas where he has not spoken. To bind the consciences of God's people to obey something God has not said can be equivalent to false prophecy. We cannot say that God has said what he did not say. I want no part of that, so I am going to be careful to interpret the Scriptures as accurately as I can and to give counsel that flows from the biblical teaching. I have no wish to bind your conscience, one way or the other, when the Scriptures do not clearly teach something.

The Path Forward

In chapter 1, I explain how marijuana works. We must understand what is actually going on when someone uses marijuana before we can move from clear biblical teaching to application regarding marijuana use. In this chapter

I will describe the cannabis plant and the complex ways it affects the user, both positive and negative. I will also explain why issues regarding a standardization of potency are difficult. Such understanding is necessary to make ethical judgments concerning cannabis use.

In chapter 2, I describe the risks involved with marijuana smoke and ingestion, including its effects on the development of the brain, immune system, and lung function, among others. When we are not given a specific biblical command, wisdom dictates that we do some sort of cost-benefit analysis to come to wise conclusions. I hope to equip you to perform that cost-benefit analysis in this chapter.

In chapter 3, I look at the relationship between the Christian and civil law. What are the issues regarding the legalization of cannabis, and is civil law a reliable guide to Christian morality? I will emphasize that the Christian is obligated to obey the law, but what the government commands, forbids, or permits is not always righteous. The Christian ultimately serves a higher authority.

Once we have established the science of how marijuana works, the risks associated with using the drug, and the legal context, we will turn to the Bible and apply what the Scriptures say about the issue of marijuana. Specifically, in chapter 4, we will look at what the Bible has to say about alcohol addiction and intoxication to determine if there are principles that apply to the use of marijuana. I will argue that though the marijuana high is different from alcohol drunkenness, the effects of drunkenness—namely, impairment of physical ability, cognitive ability, and judgment—also occur with the marijuana high, so the biblical prohibition on drunkenness applies to marijuana intoxication.

In chapter 5, I raise a series of questions related to marijuana use and Christian discipleship. Faithful followers of Jesus Christ should give due consideration to these questions. Some of them are specific to issues related to marijuana use (including marijuana use for the pleasures of getting high and marijuana use as self-medication to escape). Many of the questions could be applied to any morally indifferent issue, so the framework I am laying out can be used on a number of ethical and moral issues that the Christian will face. I hope you will go on to apply these tools in your quest to live faithfully before God.

I take up the question of medical marijuana in chapters 6 and 7. Recognizing that some doctors are now suggesting the use of marijuana for certain medical conditions and side effects, I will survey the current established science on cannabinoid use in medicine in chapter 6. We will find that while anecdotal evidence abounds, actual research is still in its early stages. Though in its infancy, this research seems to show significant medical benefits to components of the cannabis plant. Both THC and CBD have some proven medical uses.

In chapter 7, I survey the biblical teaching on what it is to be human and the biblical teaching on suffering, where it comes from, how the Lord uses it in the life of the believer, and the biblical priority on its alleviation. I then ask a series of questions designed to provide wisdom on the use of cannabis (and other mind-altering drugs) for acute suffering and for chronic suffering.

Finally, in the appendix, I bring the fruit of the content covered thus far to answer questions commonly asked by pastors and parents. This appendix will demonstrate how to apply biblical wisdom to concrete situations and will hopefully be a resource you can return to in the future after you've finished reading the book.

CHAPTER I

What Is Marijuana and How Does It Work?

Just a few blocks from my front door is the entrance to the "Green Mile" of Portland on Sandy Boulevard. Allegedly, this street has the largest concentration of cannabis dispensaries of any thoroughfare in the world. If the outrageous number of marijuana shops does not tip you off, a large billboard atop one dispensary announces that you have entered the portal to pot paradise. There are also plenty of excellent restaurants on the street that will appeal to you even if your hunger is not the product of partaking of the Green Mile's famous wares. I mean, where else can you enjoy ribs cooked up by Snoop Dog's uncle?

But you don't have to live in Portland to notice that marijuana use is on the rise.

According to *Monitoring the Future*, a long-term epidemiological study that surveys trends in legal and illicit drug use among American adolescents and adults, marijuana use in young adult men and women reached historic levels in 2019.[1] The data is summarized in the chart on the next page.

---

[1] "In general, across the years, the trends have been parallel for men and women in each age group. In the past five years (2014–2019), annual use increased 5 to 7 percentage points for men and women among nineteen- to twenty-two-year-olds (to 45% and 41%, respectively), 8 to 10 percentage points among twenty-three- to twenty-six-year-olds (to 40% and 39%), and 13 percentage points among twenty-seven- to thirty-year-olds (to 44% and 34%). The 2019 annual prevalence for men and women in each age group were at historic highs since the late 1980s." *J. E. Schulenberg et al., Monitoring the Future National Survey Results on Drug Use, 1975–2019: Volume II, College Students and Adults Ages 19–60,* vol. II (Ann Arbor, MI: Institute for Social Research, The University of Michigan, 2020), 119.

Marijuana Use Among 19–30 Years Olds in 2019[2]		
	Men	Women
Daily Use	11.5%	7.6%
Monthly Use	29.5%	24.1%
Annual Use	42.7%	39.9%

Those numbers are shockingly high. More than one in ten young adult men use marijuana daily. Teenage use is also high with 6.6 percent of eighth graders, 18.4 percent of tenth graders, and 22.3 percent of twelfth graders using marijuana over any thirty-day period.[3]

With numbers that high, the church cannot pretend its people are unaffected or do not have questions.

If you were asked what the Bible says about a topic like lying, the path to finding an answer would be straightforward. After all, the Bible has a lot to say about lying, deception, and truth. The Scriptures teach us much about God's holy character and what is found in the sinful hearts of humans. You would go to your Bible and find the places where those teachings occur. Of course, you would want to pay close attention to all the different levels of context,

---

[2] Schulenberg et al., II:57.

[3] Schulenberg et al., II:463.

being careful to understand each biblical reference according to its literary, canonical, historical, and cultural contexts. Your study would certainly take time, but the process is not terribly complicated.

When we are looking to the Scriptures for wisdom and guidance on a topic that is *not* explicitly in the Bible, the process changes. It is not a matter of going to the concordance in the back of the Bible, making a list, then taking notes on what you find when you look up each reference. Instead, you have to know something about the topic to apply the revealed wisdom we find in the Bible. Again, my conviction is that the Bible is sufficient: we have all the divine words we need to live faithfully before God in our current day (2 Tim. 3:15–16; Ps. 119:1, 9–11). That means there is sufficient wisdom and teaching in the Bible to navigate marijuana issues as well as a host of other difficult questions that require answering.

Of course, many of the decisions we make each day have no moral implications whatsoever. Such things are *adiaphora*—indifferent matters. For the most part, I do not stress over what color socks to wear in the morning or confess my poor sock choice to the Lord, even when my wife points out that my clothes do not match. Choosing between marionberry pie and German chocolate cake is really just a matter of personal preference (though why anybody would refuse to enter the after-dinner paradise of marionberry pie is beyond me).

The Bible does not come with an exhaustive account of all the things that make the "indifferent matters" list. Again, we should be grateful. Imagine trying to lug such a book full of exhaustive lists to church every Sunday. Or even worse, imagine having all 128 GB of your phone's memory filled with that data! So obviously, one of the first steps in figuring out what the Bible teaches on a specific topic is to determine whether there is any moral weight to it. And to do that, you have to know something about the thing you are investigating.

In order to understand what the Bible has to say about something that is not explicitly in the Bible, we must understand what that something is.

For example, many weighty ethical issues are not explicitly mentioned in the Scriptures—things like cloning, for example. It would be ridiculous to suggest that because cloning is not in the Bible, the Lord is indifferent to it. The Bible was written from about 1400 BC to AD 100. It was written by real people, in real languages, in a real land, in real and specific contexts. Though inspired by the Holy Spirit, the biblical authors wrote about what they knew; they addressed the issues of their day and only occasionally spoke of the future. The Bible does not mention cloning because its authors had no concept of cloning.

But the Bible does have plenty to say about such things as children, procreation, human responsibility, life, and God's sovereignty. We have to understand something about what cloning is in order to bring to bear Scripture's teaching on that difficult ethical issue.

When it comes to marijuana, many believe that we can take the Bible's teaching on alcohol and drunkenness and apply it directly to marijuana and getting high. Substitute *marijuana* for every biblical reference to *wine*; then replace *drunkenness* with the words *getting high*, and the Christian is good to go, right?

But is it actually that easy? The Bible speaks of alcohol in a variety of ways. The Scriptures are clear that drunkenness is sinful, but wine is also celebrated in the Bible and plays a vital role in the Old Testament feasts and the New Testament practice of the Lord's Supper. Further, marijuana and wine are different is some important and basic respects. Wine is a drink; marijuana is not. While both intoxicate, alcohol impacts the brain in a different manner from marijuana. A little wine does not intoxicate; it is not clear that marijuana can be smoked in moderation without effects. Therefore, simply substituting *marijuana* for *wine* will not work. To determine if we can apply the biblical teaching on alcohol and drunkenness, we must understand what marijuana is and how it works.

What Is Marijuana?

Marijuana comes from the cannabis, or hemp, plant. The most common varieties are *Cannabis sativa* and *Cannabis indica*. For many, the image of marijuana that immediately comes to mind is a green plant with long pointy leaves. There are drawings of it everywhere— T-shirts, bumper stickers, coffee mugs, even the cover of this book. Yesterday, on a walk with my wife, I saw someone wearing pants with marijuana leaf imprints. (I think they were actually pajama bottoms; my hometown is weird.) But the drug itself is a greenish-gray, sometimes brown, mixture of dried products from the cannabis plant's seeds, leaves, stems, and flowers. Resins and oils are also commonly extracted from the cannabis plant.

The dried plant products are smoked in hand-rolled cigarettes called joints (doobies, if you are over forty) or cigar wraps called blunts. Marijuana can also be smoked in water pipes called bongs. Vaping cannabis (or cannavaping) is an increasingly popular way to smoke the drug. Cannabis is often mixed into food (like brownies or candies), which are called edibles. Marijuana teas can be imbibed. The resins and oils offer a more concentrated form of the drug's active components.[4]

What Does Marijuana Do to the Brain?

The human brain is designed with microscopic sockets called cannabinoid receptors. The two main types of receptors are called CB1 and CB2. CB1 receptors are found throughout the body but are mainly concentrated in the brain and central nervous system. CB2 receptors are also found throughout the body, primarily in the immune system tissues and nerves, but can also be found in the brain. When your brain is functioning normally, neurons "communicate" with one another via chemicals called neurotransmitters. Endocannabinoids are neurotransmitters that "plug" into the cannabinoid receptors, activating those receptors, which then allows the neurons to communicate with one another. The human body creates and releases these endocannabinoids when properly stimulated. (When the human body makes them, they are called "endocannabinoids"; when they come from the cannabis plant, they are called "phytocannabinoids.") The endocannabinoids,

---

[4] "Marijuana Research Report: What Is Marijuana?" National Institute on Drug Abuse, https://www.drugabuse.gov/publications /research-reports/marijuana/what-marijuana.

cannabinoid receptors, and the enzymes that break down the endocannabinoids when they have done their job comprise the endocannabinoid system (ECS).

Scientists are still discovering what the ECS does, but it appears that it is responsible for regulating such bodily functions as appetite and digestion, metabolism, pain response, mood, sleep, the cardiovascular system, muscle formation, and many more. Many of the cannabinoid receptors are found in parts of the brain that control thinking, pleasure, concentration, coordination, time perception, and memory—basically many of the things that make you who you are and enable you to do what you do, feel what you feel, and think what you think. But the human body is not the only creator of cannabinoids.

The cannabis plant is remarkably complex, with more than four hundred chemical compounds, more than sixty of which are cannabinoids. For our purposes, the two most significant cannabinoids are Delta-9-tetrahydrocannabinol (or THC) and cannabidiol (or CBD). THC produces psychoactive effects (the "high" we associate with marijuana use), while CBD does not. For that reason, I will initially focus on THC and pick up the discussion of CBD in the medical marijuana chapters.

THC acts as an "agonist" of the cannabinoid receptors in the brain. An agonist is a molecule that mimics a biological molecule that activates receptors. When THC is so introduced, it binds to the cannabinoid receptors, producing a variety of different effects.

Marijuana acts as both a stimulant and a depressant, which explains the wide variety of effects the drug brings. THC causes, among other things, a short-lived, acute increase in dopamine levels in various parts of the brain. Dopamine is a neurotransmitter which, among other roles, is used in the pleasure pathways of the brain. The result is a general feeling of pleasure or euphoria.

For example, during pleasurable activities, such as sexual intercourse, the brain releases cannabinoids (usually a chemical called anandamide), which plug into the cannabinoid receptors, and the body responds by releasing dopamine. When the dopamine washes over your brain, you feel pleasure. Incidentally, anandamide has been found in chocolate, which might explain why virtually everybody (except one of my sons) derives pleasure from eating chocolate. There is no shame in enjoying chocolate. God designed you (and chocolate) that way.

Let's get back to THC, which is also a psychoactive cannabinoid. That is, it changes brain function and alters things such as perception and mood. The high caused by marijuana is notoriously difficult to predict because people's experiences with marijuana vary widely. But for the most part, people who are stoned have altered sensory perceptions (especially hearing and taste) and changes in their moods and mental states (for many, marijuana has a mellowing or calming effect, where situations that are neutral or potentially negative will be seen as humorous or amusing).[5]

But THC does not just bring altered perception and mood. In the hippocampus, which regulates learning and assimilating new information, THC decreases firing. The result is memory impairment and learning difficulties. In the hypothalamus, which regulates, among other things, eating, THC will increase appetite. In the cerebellum, which controls motor coordination, THC causes clumsiness and impaired coordination. In the brain stem, which regulates information between the brain and spinal column, THC will decrease nausea. The cellular reactions brought about by THC create a host of other short-term effects, including diminished problem-solving skills due to interference with frontal-executive brain function (which enables performance of tasks requiring complex thinking), increased heart rate, feelings of anxiety, panic and paranoia,

---

[5] Elizabeth Hartney, "How Marijuana Can Affect Your Mental State," *Verywell Mind*, January 6, 2020, https://www.verywellmind.com/what-does-a-marijuana-high-feel-like-22303.

altered pain sensitivity, an altered sense of the passing of time, and an overall distorted perception of reality.

What's in a Name?

Now you might infer, since these special sockets are called "cannabinoid receptors," and since the chemicals that plug into them are called "cannabinoids," that they were both specially designed to be activated by the cannabis plant. Some might even conclude that the brain functions best when cannabinoids from the cannabis plant are introduced to the brain. That inference and conclusion are absolutely false.

While it is true that cannabinoids get their name from cannabis, that is only because a group of Israeli scientists in the 1960s saw the effect of THC on certain parts of the brain before those special receptors had been named and decided to use the nomenclature "cannabinoid" to describe those receptors. Later, in the 1990s, that same team discovered why we have those receptors in the brain.[6] The name *cannabinoid* is not a testimony to design or efficiency; it is due to the timing and order of discovery.

---

[6] Elizabeth Stuyt, "The Problem with the Current High Potency THC Marijuana from the Perspective of an Addiction Psychiatrist," *Missouri Medicine* 115, no. 6 (December 2018): 482–86.

Not Your Grandfather's Ganja

Further complicating the contemporary issues surrounding marijuana use is that what was smoked during the 1960s and 1970s is not what is being consumed today. The hippie movement of the 1960s conjures up almost comical images of peaceful, loving, tie-dye-wearing young people passing around a joint, wondering why we can't give peace a chance. The hippie subculture was not always that innocuous, but even so, the marijuana consumed at the time through

> **What was smoked during the 1960s and 1970s is not what is being consumed today.**

smoking or edibles had a THC content of about 1 to 2 percent. A typical joint in the 1970s, with a THC content of 1 to 2 percent by weight, did not have near the psychoactive effects as what is smoked today and was the "cannabis equivalent of near-beer."[7] That number stayed relatively constant from the 1960s through the 1980s.

---

[7] Alex Berenson, *Tell Your Children: The Truth About Marijuana, Mental Illness, and Violence* (New York: Free Press, 2019). A shared joint with 1 to 2 percent THC by weight would result in the user inhaling about 2.5 milligrams of THC. "Cannabis advocates today generally suggest that 2.5 milligrams of THC is the equivalent of a single drink for a new or infrequent user." Ibid., 40.

Today, the latest THC content is much higher, and growers are breeding for even higher THC potency. You can walk into a cannabis dispensary and see marijuana strains with exotic names like "Laughing Buddha," "Silver Haze," and "Girl Scout Cookie" that regularly have THC contents from 17 to 25 percent, with some that exceed 30 percent.[8] These numbers refer to the marijuana that is smoked and vaped. There are also THC products such as oils and edibles with THC concentrations over 90 percent.

What about Potency?

There is currently no national industry or legal standard for marijuana potency. Where alcohol has proof (twice the alcohol percentage content by volume), there is nothing like that for marijuana for a variety of reasons. It is possible to measure the THC percentage, but there are a variety of ways to do this, and they vary from state to state. There is no national standard, and as long as marijuana remains a Schedule 1 drug (more on that in chapter 3), we should not expect one.

---

[8] Stuyt, "The Problem with the Current High Potency THC Marijuana from the Perspective of an Addiction Psychiatrist."

Further complicating the THC percentage issue is that responses to the same marijuana sample vary from person to person. With alcohol, generally speaking, it is possible to predict the impact of drinking on a person. People's responses to alcohol will be a function of body size (a large, heavy person will be able to "handle" more alcohol than a smaller, lighter person). Blood alcohol content is a reliable indicator of level of inebriation. But two people sharing the same joint will react differently, sometimes radically so.

Now that we know a little about how marijuana works and its effects on the body, we turn to the risks a Christian must consider. If the Bible does not expressly forbid marijuana use, what are the possible outcomes for partaking?

CHAPTER 2

The Risks of Marijuana Use

The other day my boys and I were driving home when we stopped at an intersection. My son, Vicente, laughing said, "Look at that sign!" A panhandler held a sign near our window that read, "I NEED WEED and FEED!" Though we chose not to contribute, we were impressed with his honesty, creativity, and Dr. Seuss-like rhyming skills. We also got to talk about how great the "need" for "weed" was in that particular street poet's life.

My young sons understood the need for "feed." Food and nutrition are a must. That is the way God designed us. But what about marijuana? Was the clever beggar exaggerating for the purpose of the rhyme, or did he actually have a biochemical or mental "need" for marijuana? Is marijuana addiction even possible?

The purpose of this chapter is to consider the risks associated with marijuana use. To this point we have established that though the Bible does not explicitly mention marijuana, because the Bible is sufficient, we have all the divine words we need in order to answer the question regarding the appropriateness of marijuana use. The goal, then, is to think like a disciple of Jesus Christ and apply the wisdom of Holy Scripture in a manner that glorifies Christ. To that end, we have to know something of the thing being considered in order to apply what Scripture teaches. We have considered the science of marijuana (what it is and how it works). Now we take up the question of what can happen to you if you use marijuana.

The question of harm or risk is important to consider because, as the apostle Paul taught, "'Everything is permissible for me,' but not everything is beneficial" (1 Cor. 6:12). Paul's words are straightforward. Christians have the liberty to engage in many different activities that are not expressly forbidden by God's Word, but just because God has not prohibited an activity does not mean it is wise to participate or partake. There are other factors to consider.

In this case, the activity might not be beneficial; that is, it might not be in your best interest. The Bible doesn't tell us exactly how to determine if something is beneficial, so I suspect there is room for disagreement. But certain or potential harm to self and others ought to be considered if one wants to avoid things that are not beneficial.

The Scriptures also teach that the human body is the temple of the Lord. Many of you are probably rolling your eyes. Perhaps your memory is flashing back to images of your mother chastising you about the evils of drinking, smoking, and chewing because, "don't you know your body is the temple of the Lord."

But here is the thing: your mother was right.

Paul taught the Christians in Corinth, "Don't you know that your body is a temple of the Holy Spirit who is in you, whom you have from God? You are not your own, for you were bought at a price. So glorify God with your body" (1 Cor. 6:19–20). There are two reasons in these two short verses Christians ought to take care of their bodies. First, our bodies are a gift from the Lord, and stewardship demands that we care for them. God may ask us to lay down our bodies for him, but that is his prerogative as Lord of our bodies.

Our bodies are a gift from the Lord, and stewardship demands that we care for them.

Second, God not only has Creator's rights over us and our bodies; he also has Redeemer's rights. Christians have been created and bought by God through the blood of Christ. Paul's conclusion is simple: God owns you; therefore honor the Lord with your body. Paul's command in 1 Corinthians 6 comes in the context of a prohibition on sexual immorality, which Paul describes as a sin against the body. Though intentionally doing things that harm the body is not exactly the same as sexual immorality, Paul's command demonstrates that what we do with our bodies matters, and care for the body and a desire to honor the Lord with our bodies are proper concerns of the Christian.

What follows in the remainder of this chapter is a discussion of the risks involved in marijuana use. It is particularly vital that we have this discussion because while marijuana use is on the rise, perception of risk is on the decline.[1]

---

[1] According to Monitoring the Future, a long-term epidemiological study that surveys trends in legal and illicit drug use among American adolescents and adults, the perceived risks of experimental, occasional, and regular marijuana use reached all-time lows among young adults (ages 19 to 30) in 2019. J. E. Schulenberg et al., *Monitoring the Future National Survey Results on Drug Use, 1975–2019: Volume II, College Students and Adults Ages 19–60*, vol. II (Ann Arbor, MI: Institute for Social Research, The University of Michigan, 2020), 9.

Is Marijuana Addictive?

A prevailing myth concerning marijuana is that it is not addictive. But that myth raises the question of what addiction is. According to the National Institute on Drug Abuse, *addiction* is defined as "a chronic, relapsing disorder characterized by compulsive drug seeking, continued use despite harmful consequences, and long-lasting changes in the brain."[2]

---

[2] "The Science of Drug Use and Addiction: The Basics," National Institute on Drug Abuse, June 25, 2020, accessed September 10, 2020, https://www.drugabuse.gov/publications/media-guide/science -drug-use-addiction-basics. The current *Diagnostic and Statistical Manual of Mental Disorders (DSM-5)*, describes a condition called "Cannabis Use Disorder." DSM-5 also describes cannabis intoxication and cannabis withdrawal, as well as cannabis-induced psychotic disorder, anxiety disorder, and sleep disorder. Cannabis use disorder occurs when marijuana use becomes problematic and is diagnosed as mild in the presence of two to three symptoms, moderate in the presence of four to five symptoms, and severe in the presence of six or more symptoms, all occurring in a twelve-month period. These symptoms include such things as simple craving, difficulty discontinuing use, tolerance, use despite harm to user, and withdrawal. Addiction is typically associated with severe substance use disorder. *Diagnostic and Statistical Manual of Mental Disorders*, 5th ed. (Arlington, VA: American Psychiatric Association, 2013), 484–519.

Studies show that 9 percent of adults and 17 percent of adolescents who use marijuana develop an addiction to it.[3] A regular user is defined as one who smokes, vapes, or consumes an edible three to four times per week. A heavy user will smoke every day of the week.[4]

Approximately one out of every ten regular users who began using as adults will develop a marijuana addiction. Significantly, more than one out of every six regular users who began using as teenagers will develop a marijuana addiction.

Now these numbers are lower than for adult addictions to nicotine, heroin, cocaine, and alcohol (32%, 23%, 17%, and 15% respectively). But "*less* addictive" does not mean "*not* addictive." The 17 percent addiction rate for adolescents is particularly troubling. As addiction consultant and professor of psychiatry Kevin P. Hill testifies,

> Our research showed that, among adolescents, progression from marijuana use

---

[3] "Is Marijuana Addictive?," National Institute on Drug Abuse, July 2, 2020, https://www.drugabuse.gov/publications/research-reports/marijuana/marijuana-addictive.

[4] Kevin P. Hill, *Marijuana: The Unbiased Truth About the World's Most Popular Weed* (Center City, MN: Hazelden Publishing, 2015), 67.

to marijuana addiction can occur very quickly and that marijuana addiction can progress to addiction of other substances very quickly as well. . . . Things can progress very quickly with addiction, especially with a brain that's still developing, and this is why *any* substance use by a young person needs to be taken as seriously as possible.[5]

Lung and Heart Issues

It should come as no surprise that the American Lung Association (ALA) is concerned about marijuana smoke being inhaled into the lungs. President Clinton once famously confessed that he had tried marijuana but did not inhale. If that were true, the risks to his lungs would have been minimized, but most marijuana users are not able to, nor are they interested in, following the president's example. Marijuana smoke is meant to be inhaled because that is the quickest route to the bloodstream. But to get to the blood, which carries the THC to the brain, the smoke

[5] Hill, *Marijuana*, 25.

must pass through the lungs first, and therein lies a big problem.

Some argue that marijuana is less dangerous than cigarette smoke, but smoke from cannabis combustion has been shown to contain many of the same toxins, irritants, and carcinogens as tobacco smoke. Pot smokers often hold the smoke in their lungs for longer periods, hoping to maximize the delivery of the THC into the bloodstream, which puts the smoker at further risk for exposure to the tar that is so harmful to the lungs.[6] The ALA warns that smoking cannabis can adversely affect the body's immune system, and it will destroy the lung's first line of defense against dust and germs.

Second-hand marijuana smoke is just as dangerous (and annoying) as secondhand tobacco smoke. The ALA's bottom-line warning is clear: "Smoking marijuana clearly damages the human lung, and regular use leads to chronic bronchitis and can cause an immune-compromised person to be more susceptible to lung infections. No one should be exposed to secondhand marijuana smoke."[7]

---

[6] "Marijuana and Lung Health," American Lung Association, May 27, 2020, https://www.lung.org/quit-smoking/smoking-facts/health-effects/marijuana-and-lung-health.

[7] Ibid.

But what about vaping? Is that less harmful to the lung than smoke? "Vaping" marijuana is done by inhaling heated up oils through an e-cigarette or a vaporizer. Vaping provides a pathway for the desired marijuana components (usually THC and CBD) without the toxins associated with the combustion of the marijuana plant. But vaping creates an entirely different problem known as "popcorn lung" or EVALI (e-cigarette or vaping product use-associated lung injury). EVALI, caused by the inhalation of vitamin E acetate, is characterized by inflammation of the lungs. The U.S. Centers for Disease Control (CDC) has designated EVALI to be a severe lung disease and reports that most EVALI cases are linked to vaping THC.[8]

Even the American Heart Association (AHA) has gotten into the game. Dr. Rose Marie Robertson, deputy chief science and medical officer for the AHA, warns, "The American Heart Association recommends that people not smoke or vape any substance, including cannabis products, because of the potential harm to the heart, lungs and

---

[8] "Outbreak of Lung Injury Associated with the Use of E-Cigarette, or Vaping Products," Centers for Disease Control and Prevention, February 25, 2020), https://www.cdc.gov/tobacco/basic_information/e-cigarettes/severe-lung-disease.html.

blood vessels."[9] The AHA believes marijuana use may be linked to an increased risk of heart attack, atrial fibrillation, tachycardia, ventricular contractions, ventricular arrhythmias, and heart failure. Further, despite the claims of some advocates, the AHA sees no cardiovascular benefits associated with marijuana use.[10]

Teen Use Interferes with Brain Development

One of the most alarming facts about marijuana is that teen and adolescent use interferes with brain development. This cannot be stressed strongly enough. THC has been proven to interfere with brain development, and the losses created by that interference cannot be restored. This is not a matter of opinion, nor is it the subjective prejudice

---

[9] "Cannabis Use Shows Substantial Risks, No Benefits for Cardiovascular Health; More Research Is Critical," American Heart Association, August 5, 2020, https://newsroom.heart.org/news/cannabis-use-shows-substantial-risks-no-benefits-for-cardiovascular-health-more-research-is-critical.

[10] Robert L. Page II et al., "Medical Marijuana, Recreational Cannabis, and Cardiovascular Health: A Scientific Statement from the American Heart Association," *Circulation* 142, no. 10 (August 5, 2020): 131–52. The American Heart Association has called for more research to be done on the cardiovascular effects of marijuana.

of a few doctors. The evidence is overwhelming, and there is no credible disagreement with that conclusion.

The human brain develops over time, with the female brain reaching peak values of brain volume earlier than males.[11] It will come as no surprise to anyone who has parented a boy, been a boy, talked to a boy, or seen a boy, that the male brain takes a bit longer to develop. This makes the young male brain particularly vulnerable to the effects of marijuana use. There is also strong evidence that the development of the prefrontal cortex of the brain, the part of the brain used by adults for rational thought and judgment, does not fully mature until the age of twenty-five.[12] This being the case, the legal limit of age twenty-one for recreational marijuana use, in those states that have taken that step, is probably too young. Brains of male users are being permanently damaged. While there is no evidence that marijuana use leads to a drop in intelligence on a fully developed adult brain (although people who are stoned are

---

[11] Rhoshel K. Lenroot and Jay N. Giedd, "Sex Differences in the Adolescent Brain," *Brain and Cognition* 72, no. 1 (November 13, 2009): 46–55, https://doi.org/10.1016/j.bandc.2009.10.008.

[12] Mariam Arain et al., "Maturation of the Adolescent Brain," *Neuropsychiatric Disease and Treatment* 9 (April 3, 2013): 449–61, https://doi.org/10.2147/NDT.S39776.

not exactly at their mental best), the evidence of damage to the immature brain is uncontested.

Dr. Madeline Meier of Duke University and her collaborators showed as much as an eight-point decline in IQ as a result of early, regular marijuana use.[13] Most people have an IQ within the range of 85 to 115 (the average is always 100), so an eight-point drop is serious. The study also showed that when the subject refrained from smoking for periods of more than a year IQ levels did *not* return to normal. Let that sink in: the IQ levels do not return to normal, even if you never smoke another joint for as long as you live.

Dr. Meier's number of an eight-point decline is hotly debated, but that a decline occurs is not debated. Her study also involved those who persistently used marijuana from a young age. So I am not saying that if teenagers smoke one joint or accidently breathe in some secondhand pot smoke, they will start dropping IQ points. But with the addictive nature of marijuana, why take the chance?

The studies linking impaired brain development with young recreational marijuana users are too numerous and

---

[13] Madeline H. Meier et al., "Persistent Cannabis Users Show Neuropsychological Decline from Childhood to Midlife," *Proceedings of the National Academy of Sciences* 109, no. 40 (October 2, 2012): E2657, https://doi.org/10.1073/pnas.1206820109.

conclusive to ignore. Dr. Jodi Gilman has shown that marijuana use is associated with brain abnormalities in young pot smokers.[14] Dr. Staci Gruber's group has demonstrated that those who smoke regularly have to use different parts of their brain to perform certain tasks.[15]

> **Studies linking impaired brain development with young recreational marijuana users are too numerous and conclusive to ignore.**

For these reasons, underage recreational marijuana use, particularly by males, is a horrible idea. To make matters worse, because the teen and young adult brain is still developing, it is even more susceptible to the effects of the drug. That susceptibility and underdeveloped brain combine to make responses to marijuana even more unpredictable, which makes the next risk I will cover even more concerning.

---

[14] Jodi M. Gilman et al., "Cannabis Use Is Quantitatively Associated with Nucleus Accumbens and Amygdala Abnormalities in Young Adult Recreational Users," *The Journal of Neuroscience* 34, no. 16 (April 16, 2014): 5529, https://doi.org/10.1523/JNEURO SCI.4745-13.2014.

[15] Staci A. Gruber et al., "Age of Onset of Marijuana Use Impacts Inhibitory Processing," *Neuroscience Letters* 511, no. 2 (2012): 89–94, https://doi.org/10.1016/j.neulet.2012.01.039.

Psychosis and Mental Illness

In 1936, the film *Reefer Madness* was released. The movie was a propaganda piece, originally financed by church groups, to demonstrate the evils and dangers of marijuana use. *Reefer Madness*, depicting marijuana users as violent, paranoid, and out of control, has since become a cult classic for its campiness and overall low quality. Today it is also used by marijuana advocates as an example of how marijuana has been demonized and its effects exaggerated. Any suggestion that there might be a tie between marijuana use and psychosis or mental illness is often dismissed by asking, "What, like in *Reefer Madness*?" I suppose the logic works something like this:

- *Reefer Madness* claimed that marijuana makes people crazy.
- *Reefer Madness* was a demonstrably bad movie.
- Therefore, marijuana does not make you crazy.

When you put it on paper like this, the argument is lousy, but there is no denying that it is still often used effectively.

Regardless of what you think of the cinematic qualities of the 1936 cult film, the reality is that a growing body of evidence links marijuana use with psychosis, mental illness, and violent behavior. The risk of psychosis is real and must be taken into consideration when thinking through the issue of marijuana use. The evidence is growing increasingly hard to ignore.

Physicians and psychologists had long suspected there was a connection between cannabis and psychosis, but the strongest definitive proof came in 1987, when Sven Andréasson was able to show that not only did marijuana use increase the risk of schizophrenia, but heightened use increased the odds of the onset of schizophrenia. The more one smoked, the greater the risk.[16] Later, in 2002, scientists from New Zealand found that people who had used marijuana by age fifteen were four times more likely to be diagnosed with

> A growing body of evidence links marijuana use with psychosis, mental illness, and violent behavior.

---

[16] S. Andréasson et al., "Cannabis and Schizophrenia. A Longitudinal Study of Swedish Conscripts," *Lancet* 2, no. 8574 (December 26, 1987): 1483–86, https://doi.org/10.1016/s0140-6736(87)92620-1.

schizophreniform disorder and depression by the age of twenty-six.[17]

Since that time, study after study has been performed, showing that marijuana use increases the risk for psychosis in general and schizophrenia in particular. One study in Great Britain demonstrated that using marijuana five times or more increased the risk of psychotic disorders by a factor of almost seven,[18] while another showed that teenage marijuana use tripled the risk of late-onset psychosis.[19] The list could go on and on.[20]

---

[17] Louise Arseneault et al., "Cannabis Use in Adolescence and Risk for Adult Psychosis: Longitudinal Prospective Study," *BMJ (Clinical Research Ed.)* 325, no. 7374 (November 23, 2002): 1212–13, https://doi.org/10.1136/bmj.325.7374.1212.

[18] Antti Mustonen et al., "Adolescent Cannabis Use, Baseline Prodromal Symptoms and the Risk of Psychosis," *The British Journal of Psychiatry* 212, no. 4 (April 2018): 227–33, https://doi.org/10.1192/bjp.2017.52.

[19] Hannah J. Jones et al., "Association of Combined Patterns of Tobacco and Cannabis Use in Adolescence with Psychotic Experiences," *JAMA Psychiatry* 75, no. 3 (March 1, 2018): 240–46, https://doi.org/10.1001/jamapsychiatry.2017.4271.

[20] For both a summary of the scientific evidence and an explanation as to why the evidence is largely ignored in America, please read Alex Berenson, *Tell Your Children: The Truth About Marijuana, Mental Illness, and Violence* (New York: Free Press, 2019). See especially chapter 8, pages 120–27.

Between 2000 and 2015, Dr. Brad Roberts studied the data from hospital emergency rooms in Colorado, the first state to legalize marijuana in 2012. Based on the numbers analyzed, Roberts concluded,

> Cannabis legalization has led to significant health consequences, particularly to patients in emergency departments and hospitals in Colorado. The most concerning include psychosis, suicide, and other substance abuse. Deleterious effects on the brain include decrements in complex decision-making, which may not be reversible with abstinence. Increases in fatal motor vehicle collisions, adverse effects on cardiovascular and pulmonary systems, inadvertent pediatric exposures, cannabis contaminants exposing users to infectious agents, heavy metals, and pesticides, and hash-oil burn injuries in preparation of drug concentrates have been documented.[21]

---

[21] Brad A. Roberts, "Legalized Cannabis in Colorado Emergency Departments: A Cautionary Review of Negative Health and Safety

That is quite a list, and while there may be other contributing factors to the increases cited in the report, awareness and caution are certainly in order.

The evidence linking marijuana use and psychosis is too great to ignore and must be taken into account when trying to decide whether or not to use the drug. I would think that if a person comes from a family with a history of mental illness, he should be wary of cannabis or any THC product.

There is also evidence that marijuana use increases violent behavior. This seems strange because we associate being high with being mellow and calm. Getting stoned and getting violent is counterintuitive. But we must remember that people often respond to THC in radically different ways. And if marijuana causes psychotic episodes, then its causing violent behavior is not that surprising.

One study published in the *Journal of Interpersonal Violence* shows that consistent adolescent marijuana use nearly doubles the risk of committing domestic violence by the age of twenty-six.[22] Another study of travelers in Europe showed that marijuana use doubled the risk of

Effects," *The Western Journal of Emergency Medicine* 20, no. 4 (July 2019): 557–72, https://doi.org/10.5811/westjem.2019.4.39935.

[22] Jennifer M Reingle et al., "The Relationship between Marijuana Use and Intimate Partner Violence in a Nationally Representative,

fighting.[23] Investigative reporter and author Alex Berenson claims, "Over and over, (studies) have found marijuana use or abuse is strongly associated with violence—more strongly than alcohol, in many cases."[24] Will you become violent if you start smoking pot or consuming edibles? Probably not, but maybe. The risk must be taken into consideration.

Other Potential Problems

Risk of addiction, brain development interference, lung and heart problems, psychosis, and violence make up quite a list of risks. But other problems associated with marijuana use should also be considered.

Here's a fun one: cannabinoid hyperemesis syndrome, AKA "uncontrollable nausea and vomiting." Gross. Even though THC has been proven to act against nausea, heavy marijuana users (approximately ten times per day—most

---

Longitudinal Sample," *Journal of Interpersonal Violence* 27, no. 8 (May 2012): 1562–78, https://doi.org/10.1177/0886260511425787.

[23] Karen Hughes et al., "Predictors of Violence in Young Tourists: A Comparative Study of British, German and Spanish Holidaymakers," *European Journal of Public Health* 18 (October 1, 2008): 569–74, https://doi.org/10.1093/eurpub/ckn080.

[24] Berenson, *Tell Your Children: The Truth About Marijuana, Mental Illness, and Violence*, 167.

would call it an overdose) occasionally develop this syndrome.

In 2018, the American Academy of Pediatrics also gave stern warnings against marijuana use during pregnancy.[25] Consuming cannabis during pregnancy has been determined to result in lower birth rates. Both THC and CBD could have an adverse effect on the mother and the child in utero. This warning is troubling when you consider that marijuana is widely touted for nausea relief. The study cited above also raises concerns about the use of marijuana while breastfeeding.

Finally, psychologists have also determined that regular marijuana use has a negative effect on personal ambition. Of course, this fits the common stereotype of a user: stoned twenty-something men, living in their parents' basements, smoking their lives away. Doctors and psychologists call it amotivational syndrome, and it has been proven to correlate with regular marijuana use.[26] What is

---

[25] Sheryl A. Ryan, Seth D. Ammerman, and Mary E. O'Connor, "Marijuana Use During Pregnancy and Breastfeeding: Implications for Neonatal and Childhood Outcomes," *Pediatrics* 142, no. 3 (September 1, 2018): e20181889, https://doi.org/10.1542/peds .2018-1889.

[26] Andrew Lac and Jeremy Luk, "Testing the Amotivational Syndrome: Marijuana Use Longitudinally Predicts Lower

interesting is that scientists can now explain why. It turns out that THC impairs episodic memory and episodic foresight.[27] Episodic memory enables you to recollect previous experiences and put them in the proper context. Episodic

Regular marijuana use has a negative effect on personal ambition.

foresight enables you to project yourself into the future and imagine situations and outcomes. Regular marijuana users can't remember what worked in the past, nor can they simulate future actions with desired outcomes. Without these two cognitive abilities, goal creation is all but impossible. Seeing past that last bag of Doritos becomes pretty challenging.

So those are some of the risks. True, not all these possible bad outcomes are going to happen to every marijuana user. But some of them can happen. If you fit the right profile (e.g., a teenager, genetically predisposed to some

Self-Efficacy Even After Controlling for Demographics, Personality, and Alcohol and Cigarette Use. Prev Sci. 2018;19(2):117-126.," *Prev Sci* 19, no. 2 (February 2018): 117–26, https://doi.org/doi:10.1007/s11121-017-0811-3.

[27] Kimberly Mercuri et al., "Episodic Foresight Deficits in Regular, but Not Recreational, Cannabis Users," *Journal of Psychopharmacology* 32, no. 8 (June 13, 2018): 876–82, https://doi.org/10.1177/0269881118776672.

of the outcomes, a pregnant woman, etc.), the odds are frightening. If you are contemplating marijuana use, you need to ask yourself, "Is it worth the risk to myself and to others?"

CHAPTER 3

The Christian and the Law

One summer in the 1980s, I attended the Coos County Fair in my small South Coast Oregon hometown of Myrtle Point. At one point I found myself in the exhibition hall, where I passed a booth promoting the legalization of marijuana. The person manning the booth certainly looked the part of a marijuana advocate, a mid-eighties version of a West Coast hippie. Not the least bit interested in the cause, I rushed past, hoping to avoid eye contact with the activist and the awkward conversation that would inevitably follow.

Apparently I didn't move fast enough because he politely asked me to sign the petition. I remember my response, not because of my boldness or moral eloquence but more because of my rudeness. "Oh, no. I could never sign that," I dismissed him while walking quickly away. *I was a Christian*, after all. And it was self-evident, at least to me, that Christians could never support the legalization of marijuana.

Mind you, I would not have been able to give any biblical reasons for my position. If pressed, I might have mumbled something about our bodies being the temple of God and it would be wrong to "pollute" them with such a "foul" substance. I could not have told you why the substance was so "foul" or what it would do to "pollute" the temple of the living God. When it came down to it, I believed marijuana was wrong because it was against the law. If it's against the law, it is bad, and if it's legal, it is good—or at least okay. Without knowing it, I had equated the civil law of our land with the moral will of God.

The Law of God and Civil Law

There might have been a time when the Christian could lazily look to the civil law of the land as a guide to what is good and right. If those days ever existed (which I seriously doubt), they are certainly over now.

But what should the relationship be between the follower of Christ and the civil law of the land? To determine what the Scriptures have to say about marijuana and the Christian, we need to think first about the relationship between the Christian and civil (federal, state, local) government.

The clearest biblical teaching on the Christian and government is found in Romans 13.

> Let everyone submit to the governing authorities, since there is no authority except from God, and the authorities that exist are instituted by God. So then, the one who resists the authority is opposing God's command, and those who oppose it will bring judgment on themselves. For rulers are not a terror to good conduct, but to bad. Do you want to be unafraid of the one in authority? Do what is good, and you will have its approval. For it is God's servant for your good. But if you do wrong, be afraid, because it does not carry the sword for no reason. For it is God's servant, an avenger that brings wrath on the one who does wrong. Therefore, you must submit, not only because of wrath but also because

of your conscience. And for this reason you pay taxes, since the authorities are God's servants, continually attending to these tasks. Pay your obligations to everyone: taxes to those you owe taxes, tolls to those you owe tolls, respect to those you owe respect, and honor to those you owe honor. (vv. 1–7)

Here, the apostle Paul teaches that Christians are to submit to governing authorities, and they are to do so for three important reasons.

First, the authority the government wields is derived from God himself. The Bible begins with the teaching, "In the beginning God created the heavens and the earth" (Gen. 1:1). This passage is so familiar that we often forget that it teaches some of the most foundational truths in the entire Bible. Before there was anything, God already existed. In the beginning God already was. "Was what?" you might ask. We don't know. We just know he was already "there," wherever and whatever "there" is before creation.

Then God created, and all else, apart from God, came into existence. This means two kinds of things exist. There is God and the stuff God made. If you are God, then you are not something that was made. If you are something that was made, then you are not God.

In theology we call this the "Creator-creature distinction." In short form it is this: *God is God and you are not.* We might think this is so obvious that it need not be said, but if you walk down one of the more strange streets in my hometown (city motto: Keep Portland Weird!), you will run into many people to whom the Creator-creature distinction is not so obvious. When we get the Creator-creature distinction wrong, when we ignore the teachings of the first verse of the Bible, we are going to go sideways immediately.

There are many implications to the Creator-creature distinction, but for our purposes the most important is this: like all creators, God has creator's rights over what he has made. And since he made all things, he has authority over all things. In Romans 13, Paul teaches that the governmental authorities exist because God, the one who possesses all authority, has "instituted" them (Rom. 13:1). That is, government exists because God has ordained it, and government has authority because God has delegated his authority to it.

Government is a good gift from God. Recall Romans 13:2: "The one who resists the authority is opposing God's command." Unless otherwise instructed, to disobey the government is to disobey God. This means that it should be the initial impulse, the automatic reflex of Christians, to obey their governmental authorities.

Second, it is in our best interest to obey the government. Again, Paul was clear about this. Government is "God's servant for your good" (v. 4). So there are pragmatic reasons for submitting to governmental authority. Government is the generous and good provision of the Lord, intended for our protection and well-being. Generally speaking, if you want things to go well for you, submit to your governmental authority.

Unless otherwise instructed, to disobey the government is to disobey God.

Third, disobeying the government will result in judgment. This reason is the converse of the second. Because governmental authority is delegated from God, there are penalties for disobedience. I don't have to tell you that governmental authority can be coercive. Anybody who has run afoul of the law knows this full well. The government has the power to inflict penalties upon those who do not submit. It carries "the sword." Therefore, we must understand the government's authority to inflict those penalties to be ordained by God. Government acts as God's "avenger" bringing "wrath" (v. 4). If you want to live peaceably, obey the government. If you want to live under the threat of punishment, disobey the government.[1]

Paul concludes by drawing out some implications of what he has just taught. If all government is ordained by God, then we must honor our governmental authorities as such (vv. 6–7). The church desperately needs this teaching in today's bitter and caustic political climate. We must remember that Paul most likely wrote these instructions to the church in Rome when Nero sat upon the imperial throne. Virtually no credible historian, secular or Christian, thinks Nero was anything other than chaotic and maniacal—an emperor so evil that he makes most contemporary governmental leaders seem angelic in comparison. So we can't get off the hook from giving our officials honor and respect through an appeal to our special circumstances.

I fear that Christians are often in violation of these biblical commands to honor and respect our leaders (v. 7). From the cowardly confines of social media, it seems that Christians feel a carte blanche freedom to blast away at our leaders without godly restraint. Name calling, imprecations, cursing, mocking, and ridicule flow easily from the

---

[1] This is what made the civil rights movement of the 1960s so powerful. Those leading the civil rights movement knew that the government carried this power and were willing to peaceably face the consequences for their righteous disobedience.

mouths and social media accounts of Christians. We ought to remember the example of the archangel Michael "who did not dare utter a slanderous condemnation against (the devil) but said, 'The Lord rebuke you!'" (Jude 9). Let that sink in. Jude was talking about the devil! Despite the rhetoric of our current political climate, surely none of our elected officials or candidates (all of whom bear the image of God) have sunk to the level of Satan himself.

Human Government Doesn't Always Get It Right

All this is *not* to say that governmental authorities, by virtue of their ordained position and delegated authority, are automatically above reproach. Paul nuances his commands by saying we are to give honor and respect to those *to whom we owe honor and respect.* Part of our civic duty in a constitutional republic with democratic privileges and responsibilities is to vote and question our leaders, keeping them accountable for their actions. But such responsibility is to be exercised in a manner befitting a disciple of Jesus Christ. We should not let Paul's nuance act as a catchall reason to disrespect our authorities merely because we disagree with them. Throughout the rest of this chapter, where we will explore the limits of civil law, we must bear that responsibility to exhibit respect.

So government exists by the ordination of God, exercising an authority that is delegated by God. But government is *not* God. Civil government is made up of humans, all of whom, sharing common ancestry with Adam and Eve, are fallen and sinful, prone to error and overreach. Therefore, the government will occasionally prescribe things that are wrong and forbid things that are good. When the government does that, because its authority is delegated and not inherent, it has exceeded its limits, thereby losing its moral authority. In such cases the Christian is not obligated to obey.

We must remember that there may be a price to pay for disobeying civil authority. The government, however flawed, still possesses "the sword," which it will use to coerce obedience.

What the government commands is not always righteous, and the Christian is not obligated to obey the government by disobeying God. We see in texts such as Daniel 1:8; 3:16–18; and 6:10, that faithful followers of God must not obey commands that contravene the law of God. In these cases hostile governments had required the exiled Israelites to defile themselves by eating unclean foods, worshipping idols, and praying only to the king of Persia, respectively. The clearest statement in the Scriptures of the principle lived out by Daniel and his friends is found in

Acts 4 when the apostles found themselves sideways with the Jewish leadership. The authorities forbade them from preaching Jesus, to which Peter responded, "Whether it's right in the sight of God for us to listen to you rather than to God, you decide; for we are unable to stop speaking about what we have seen and heard" (Acts 4:19–20).

> **What the government commands is not always righteous, and the Christian is not obligated to obey the government by disobeying God.**

So occasionally, Christians will have to stand in opposition to their human governments.

Further, what the government defines as lawful is not always appropriate for the believer. The government allows many activities the Bible describes as sinful. Sometimes the government just gets it wrong. For example, sex outside the covenant marriage relationship between one man and one woman is forbidden by God and yet allowed by civil governments (for the most part). Drunkenness is a sin, but unless you leave the confines of your home and/or get behind the wheel, government (for the most part) doesn't care. Jim Crow laws used to be the standard in most American states, but the government got it inexcusably wrong. Racism is a repudiation of the gospel of Jesus Christ.

Sometimes the government has no business writing God's moral code into the civil law of the land. Gluttony is clearly a sin, but the civil government (thankfully) is not interested in prosecuting uncontrolled eating. And these are just sins of action. Consider also that the Bible names sins of the heart as well. Who wants to live in a land whose civil government prosecutes such things as lust, envy, or pride? Governments are not called or competent to exercise that level of moral oversight.

Civil law is not a reliable indicator of what God approves or of what he disapproves.

What does all of this have to do with the marijuana issue? Looking to the government to define good and evil, what is wise and profitable and what is not, is a bad idea. Civil law is not a reliable indicator of what God approves or of what he disapproves. The Christian is going to have to dig deeper into God's laws to make such judgments.

The Laws Regarding Marijuana

Regarding marijuana, what is the law of the land?

Ever since 1937, when President Franklin D. Roosevelt signed into federal law the Marihuana Tax

Act, the possession and sale of cannabis, for any purpose, including medical, has effectively been against federal law. One could register (by paying registration and annual fees) to buy marijuana for medical, research, and industrial purposes. That law levied a tax of $100/ounce (in 1937 dollars) for the sale of marijuana to anyone who had not registered and paid the annual fee. The tax was lower, but still prohibitive, when selling to registered buyers. In the 1950s congress passed mandatory sentencing for cannabis possession.

In 1969, the U.S. Supreme Court determined the Tax Act of 1937 to be unconstitutional. Congress responded by repealing the mandatory sentencing laws and passing the Controlled Substances Act in 1970, and marijuana was classified as a Schedule 1 substance. Schedule 1 drugs, according to the U.S. Drug Enforcement Agency (DEA) have "no currently accepted medical use in the United States, a lack of accepted safety for use under medical supervision, and a high potential for abuse."[2] More man-

---

[2] U.S. Department of Justice, Drug Enforcement Administration, "Controlled Substance Schedules," https://www.deadiversion.usdoj .gov/schedules/index.html. In addition to marijuana, the list of Schedule 1 drugs includes heroin, LSD, peyote, methaqualone ("Quaalude"), and 3,4-methylenedioxymethamphetamine (commonly referred to as "MDMA" or "Ecstasy").

datory sentencing laws were passed during the Reagan Administration of the 1980s, including the three-strikes law, which required a mandatory twenty-five-year prison sentence for repeated serious crimes, including drug offenses. Though states have attempted to bypass the federal restrictions, the U.S. Congress and Supreme Court have resisted following the lead of the states. The Obama administration's policy was to discourage U.S. attorneys from enforcing federal law against activities that were legal according to the laws of individual states. Later the Trump administration rescinded that policy.

The bottom line: as of 2020, it was still a violation of federal law to use, possess, or sell marijuana of any kind (both recreational and medical).

So, what is going on in the states that are legalizing medical and recreational marijuana? The situation is dynamic, so a list will certainly be outdated shortly after compiling it. Marijuana advocacy groups have typically followed a pattern of first, decriminalization, followed by medical marijuana legalization, and finally recreational marijuana legalization. Decriminalization means that marijuana possession will not involve criminal prosecution or arrest but will result in a smaller civil penalty (much like a traffic violation). As of the date of this writing, the following was true of states and their marijuana laws:

- Marijuana was fully legal (recreational and medical) in seventeen states and the District of Columbia.
- Recreational marijuana was decriminalized and medical marijuana was allowed in twelve states.
- Medical marijuana was legal, though recreational marijuana had not been decriminalized in seven states.
- Recreational marijuana was decriminalized, but medical marijuana was not legal in one state (though CBD oil was allowed for medicinal purposes in that state).
- Recreational marijuana was not decriminalized, and medical marijuana was not legal in six states (though CBD oil was allowed for medicinal purposes in all six).
- Marijuana of any kind was completely illegal in eight states (though it had been decriminalized in two of those states).[3]

---

[3] "Map of Marijuana Legality by State," DISA, https://disa.com /map-of-marijuana-legality-by-state.

Oregon was the first state to decriminalize small amounts of marijuana in 1973, just three years after passage of the Federal Controlled Substance Act. Medical marijuana was first legalized in California in 1996. Colorado and Washington were the first states to legalize recreational marijuana in 2012. The changes to legalization of medical and recreational marijuana at the state level have taken place during the lifetimes of most of the people reading this book. There is currently a strong push to remove marijuana from the list of Schedule 1 drugs. Unless something drastically changes in public perception, marijuana advocacy has a momentum that is most likely going to eventuate in federal legalization and acceptance in all fifty states in America.

Marijuana advocacy has a momentum that is most likely going to eventuate in federal legalization and acceptance in all fifty states in America.

Assessing Intoxication

Every state in the union has strict laws against driving under the influence of intoxicants (DUII). Assessing intoxication caused by marijuana use is notoriously difficult. Many people just assume that intoxication from alcohol and intoxication from marijuana are effectively the same thing, so detection of the two would be the same. That is, since a Breathalyzer can be used to determine blood alcohol content, can't the same be done for marijuana? Unfortunately, determining THC levels in the body requires a blood draw, and critics are concerned that the results are too imprecise.

Unlike alcohol, which has only one intoxicating component (ethanol) that is *not* stored in the body, marijuana has many psychoactive components. Further, some THC from marijuana use is immediately stored in the fat cells of the body and is released slowly over time. For this reason, a person who used marijuana one day might have THC detected in his blood three weeks later. THC stays in the bloodstream for a long time, even when the "high" does not. Stories abound of users who have failed an employee blood test but swear they had not used the drug for weeks.

Even though recreational and/or medical marijuana might be legal in your state, that does not mean your employer will accept its use. A failed drug test might be grounds for dismissal or the refusal to extend an employment contract, even in states where cannabis consumption is legal.

Establishing inebriation and impairment levels for marijuana use has been challenging. Some states have placed limits on THC blood levels. Some states, particularly those where marijuana has not been legalized, have a zero-tolerance policy, and any detected THC in the blood will result in arrest. Other states rely on field sobriety tests to determine impairment.

So the stakes for the Christian are high. Remember that civil law is not a reliable indicator of what is right or wrong, wise or foolish. Even if it were, all of these issues combined make for a complex, confusing reality.

When it comes to marijuana, the church in most places across America is no longer able to simply make an appeal to civil prohibition and be done with the question. Christians are going to have to (dare I say it?) think like disciples of Jesus Christ. And maybe that's a good thing.

CHAPTER 4

The Bible and Marijuana

After doing a presentation at a church, a middle-aged man approached me to ask if I would listen to a specific biblical argument. I replied that I was always willing to listen to an argument from the Scriptures, so he proceeded.

"Didn't God give to Adam every tree, plant, and herb for his good?" he asked.

"Yes, that is what the Bible says in Genesis 2." I answered.

"So, how can you say marijuana is bad?" he reasoned.

"Well, I didn't actually say marijuana is bad. I said that it can be misused. Kind of like hemlock. God made it, but it can be misused."

"But hemlock is a poison. And besides, God put the tree of life in the garden of Eden. And isn't another name for marijuana 'tree'? So marijuana must be good." (He was serious.)

This line of argumentation has been repeated to me multiple times. Ironically, the same logic is used to argue against marijuana. I have had people tell me, "Another name for marijuana is 'weed,' and we all know that weeds are a result of the curse after the fall in Genesis 3."

Tree and *weed* are slang terms for marijuana, and neither trace back to biblical times. Though those two words are found in English translations of the Bible, they don't refer to the cannabis plant. The word *pot* appears in many English translations, but no one would argue that references to kettles in the Bible are simultaneously affirming the use of marijuana. On that same note, there is a popular strain of marijuana called "Angel OG." Users might be hopeful, but there is no angelic origin to that particular plant. English slang terms provide little to no insight, so nothing is to be gained by studying their origins.

Despite attempts by both advocates and critics to find marijuana in the Bible, there are no biblical references to the cannabis plant. To gain wisdom from the Scriptures on the topic of marijuana, we can't just turn to the concordance in the back of our Bibles and look hopefully for references to marijuana or cannabis.

We have to start at the beginning if we are going to understand what Scripture has to say about anything, much less marijuana. And by the beginning, I mean the very beginning, the beginning of the Bible and everything else.

Genesis 1:1 tells us, "In the beginning God created the heavens and the earth." Much like "from A to Z," "heavens and earth" functions as what is called a *merism*, the listing of the extreme parts to represent the whole. In this case,

The Bible: God Is a Good Creator

when the author of Genesis says God created the heavens and the earth, he is saying God created everything.

On the third day God created the plants of the earth. "Then God said, 'Let the earth produce vegetation: seed-bearing plants and fruit trees on the earth bearing fruit with seed in it according to their kinds.' And it was so" (v. 11). After creating the first man and woman, he told them, "Look, I have given you every seed-bearing plant on the surface of the entire earth and every tree whose fruit contains seed. This will be food for you, for all the wildlife of the earth, for every bird of the sky, and for every creature that crawls on the earth—everything having the breath of life in it—I have given every green plant for food" (vv. 29–30). God's assessment of the plants he had just made was that they were "good." This appraisal occurred at the end of each day, and his evaluation of all that he had made when his creative work was finished was that it was "very good indeed" (v. 31).

Trouble entered paradise almost immediately. The man and the woman rebelled against their good Creator, introducing sin into the world. Interestingly, that sin involved the misuse of a plant. Eve, followed almost immediately by her husband, Adam, decided to disregard the instructions of the Lord, eating from the tree of the knowledge of good and evil. God judged the first man and woman with physical death and immediate spiritual death, separation from God when they were driven from the garden, and punishments related to who they were as male and female. Of particular interest is the curse brought against the man:

> And he said to the man, "Because you lis-
> tened to your wife and ate from the tree
> about which I commanded you, 'Do not
> eat from it':
> The ground is cursed because of you.
> You will eat from it by means of painful
>   labor

all the days of your life.
It will produce thorns and thistles for
    you,
and you will eat the plants of the field.
You will eat bread by the sweat of your
    brow
until you return to the ground,
since you were taken from it.
For you are dust,
and you will return to dust."
(Gen. 3:17–19)

A few focused observations are in order.

First, God made the plants. And that includes *Cannabis sativa*, *Cannabis indica*, and all the other varieties of the cannabis plants. I suppose we could speculate that the cannabis plant is the product of the curse, part of the "thorns and thistles" that would grow whenever Adam in the post-fall world tried to work the land. But I think that speculation is unfounded.

God said that work for Adam was going to be difficult and "thorns and thistles" were going to spring up where and when they were not wanted, like when Adam was trying to grow, say, grapes or wheat. Besides, even thorns and thistles have benefits. I know people who swear by taking stinging nettle pills. Stinging nettle! (I don't know who intentionally first put that nasty plant into their mouth, hoping it had health benefits, but someone apparently did.) So, unless we want to assert that cannabis is a product of the fall, an assertion that is impossible to back up from Scripture, we must acknowledge God's creation of the cannabis plant.

Second, not only did God make everything, but everything he made was good. Christians who believe the Bible are to understand that the material world is good. There is no room in the Christian worldview for some sort of second-class status for the material in contrast to the spiritual. The earth and all that it contains, including our bodies and plants, are good. They are the good and direct creation of God. As the cannabis plant is part of that creation, Christians must acknowledge that the cannabis plant is good.

But what did God mean by "good"? The Hebrew word translated "good" is *tob* (pronounced "tove"). Much like *good* in English, *tob* is a fluid word with a wide variety of possible meanings but (usually) only one meaning in context. Sometimes *tob* has a strong moral meaning (e.g., "Being kind is a good thing to do"); other times *tob* is a judgment of effectiveness or utility (e.g., "That's a good tool for the job"). Both senses are found in Genesis 2:9.

"The LORD God caused to grow out of the ground every tree pleasing in appearance and good for food, including the tree of life in the middle of the garden, as well as the tree of the knowledge of good and evil." "Good for food" speaks to effective utility; "good and evil" speaks to moral content. What can we conclude about God's appraisal of all that he made as "very good, indeed"? Primarily, it carries an effi-

> God's creation was exactly what God wanted. It worked. And, since the world was created by God, it certainly was not evil.

cient utility. God's creation was exactly what God wanted. It worked. And, since the world was created by God, it certainly was not evil.

Third, God made the plants and gave them to humans for food (and we must assume other uses) before the fall of Genesis 3. A strong theme of the creation narrative is that God is generous. In Genesis 2:8, we are told that God "planted a garden in Eden" and placed the man there in the garden to "work it and watch over it" (Gen. 2:8, 15). God also famously planted two trees in the garden: the tree of life and the tree of the knowledge of good and evil (Gen. 2:9). We should understand even these trees to be the generous provision of a benevolent God. There is no reason to think God planted a good garden and the serpent snuck in and planted a morally evil tree in the middle of paradise.

For the record, there is no biblical reason to claim that cannabis is the tree of life or the tree of the knowledge of good and evil. In fact, there is good biblical reason to deny this is the case. Despite the hopeful speculations of marijuana advocates, we have to admit that those two trees were fruit trees. When Eve ate from the tree of the knowledge of good and evil, she "took some of its fruit and ate it" (Gen. 3:6). The text does not say, "Eve harvested some leaves and quickly baked up some marijuana brownies (the first cannabis edibles!). She ate some of the brownies and also gave some to her husband, who was with her, and he ate them." That story may be funny, but it's not biblical.

Fourth, it is possible to misuse God's good creation. In fact, the sin of Adam and Eve was precisely that—the misuse of a plant God had put in the garden. The presence of the tree of the knowledge of good and evil was not the problem; nor did Adam and Eve sin by looking at the tree or touching it. Their sin was in doing what God had forbidden—eating from the tree.

All this leads me to the following conclusions about cannabis:

Cannabis is the good provision of a kind and benevolent God. It is not inherently evil. The cannabis plant is a remarkably complex plant with many components. When we discuss medical marijuana in chapter 6, we will see some of the good uses for some of those components. I don't think scientists have even scratched the surface of what cannabis can do.

Hemp, a variety of *Cannabis sativa*, enjoys a strong history in America. It has been a cash crop since at least the early 1600s and was used for paper, fabric, and rope. (The word *canvas* derives from the Latin *cannabis*.) Presidents George Washington and Thomas Jefferson grew hemp on their plantations. Hemp seeds are a valuable source of the CBD component (more on CBD in chapter 6) and of nutrition. Hemp was an American staple until 1937 when the Marihuana Tax Act effectively ended the industry. There are plenty of

> **The Bible may not mention marijuana specifically, but it has a lot to say about addiction and intoxication.**

good uses for the cannabis plant. We should be grateful to the Lord for his kind provision.

Cannabis, like any of the Lord's good gifts, can be misused. There are probably many ways to misuse marijuana, but the primary ways, the ways most interesting to readers of this book, are addiction and intoxication. The Bible may not mention marijuana specifically, but it has a lot to say about addiction and intoxication.

The Bible: Is Addiction Wrong?

Earlier we looked at the first phrase of 1 Corinthians 6:12 and Paul's teaching that not everything that is permitted is beneficial. I argued that one way to determine whether something is beneficial is to consider the risks associated with that activity. Let's take a deeper look at that passage.

> "Everything is permissible for me," but
> not everything is beneficial. "Everything
> is permissible for me," but I will not be
> mastered by anything. (1 Cor. 6:12)

Paul taught in verse 12 that though many things are permissible, it is possible to be mastered by those things. "Things" here could be literally anything, anything that is permitted—engaging in an activity or consuming a substance like food, drink, and yes, even marijuana. Christians have the liberty to engage in all sorts of activities, but that does not mean those activities are necessarily good. One test for whether something is good, according to Paul, is to ask the question, "Will this activity master me?" or "Will this activity enslave me?"

Paul's logic in the passage is straightforward. The Christian has been created and bought by the Lord, and it is God's prerogative, not ours, to exercise lordship over us (1 Cor. 6:19–20). Our bodies belong to him. It is the Lord's right to direct what we do with our bodies. It is not our right, and it is certainly not the right of an activity or substance.

To be mastered by an activity or substance is to deny the lordship of Jesus Christ. We earlier defined *addiction* as "compulsive substance use or behavior despite self-harm or negative consequences." We see how addiction fits into what Paul prohibited in 1 Corinthians 6. If we are willing to risk harm to self or others because our compulsion to consume a substance is so great, then that substance—alcohol or marijuana or anything else—has enslaved us. It is exercising a mastery over us that rightfully belongs only to Jesus Christ.

> To be mastered by an activity or substance is to deny the lordship of Jesus Christ.

Let's be specific about marijuana. If your desire for marijuana is so great that you risk harm to self or others in order to use the drug, then you have been mastered by marijuana. That self-harm could be such things as missing appointments, failing to keep your word, lying to cover up your marijuana use, refusing to commit to a job or school, stealing money to feed your habit, eating your little brother's Hostess Twinkies without permission, or spending money on pot that was budgeted (or should have been budgeted) for other things. If any of this describes your behavior when using marijuana, then it has assumed a lordship role in your life that is reserved for Jesus Christ. You are addicted and that is sin.

The Bible: Is Alcohol Use Wrong?

I have a confession to make. Though I live in Southeast Portland, perhaps the hipster capital of the world, there is nothing about me that is hipsteresque. I don't even pretend to be one. Consider the following evidence: I am absolutely incapable of growing a beard, and you would have to hit me in the head with a shovel before I would put on a pair of skinny jeans. I have no piercings on my body of any kind (aside from the self-inflicted wounds caused by stepping on my boys' Lego blocks). I have no artwork on my body at all. Frankly, I can't think of a message I want to imprint on my body that will still be insightful one month from now, let alone for the rest of my life. And my arms are so skinny that any inked message would have to be an abbreviated memo, at best. I don't like the taste of coffee, and though I live in an area famous for its craft beer, I don't enjoy alcohol at all. I really don't know how I have survived in this town for so long. It can only be the Trail Blazers and the food trucks.

Seriously, I am effectively a teetotaler. My grandfather was an alcoholic and died of liver failure. My mother grew up in that devastating environment and subsequently had little patience with alcohol consumption. It was not around our house at all.

But my conviction is that alcohol is a gift from the Lord, a gift that can be and is often misused but a gift nonetheless. There is too much in the Bible to suggest otherwise. Thus, I don't seek to bind the consciences of other believers with my personal decision about alcohol.

Wine plays a vital role in biblical theology. It is evidence of the Lord's blessing (Isa. 55:1; Joel 2:19–24; Amos 9:13–14; Ps. 104:14–15), while a lack of wine is evidence of God's judgment (Jer. 48:33; Hosea 2:9). The drink offering of wine was part of the sacrificial system under the Mosaic Covenant (Exod. 29:38–40). Wine was part of the Passover ritual and was then incorporated into the Lord's Supper (Luke 22:14–22; 1 Cor. 11:25–26). The psalmist's positive assessment of wine is that it "makes human hearts glad" (Ps. 104:14–15). Jesus had a reputation for enjoying wine (Matt. 11:19) and made some for his first public miracle (John 2:1–12). Alcohol even has some medicinal value (1 Tim. 5:23). Wine plays a significant role in the promised consummation of the kingdom of God with Christ (Matt. 26:29).

But all of that is consistent with what I just said about all the things the Lord has made. Alcohol is a gift from the Lord, but it can be misused and abused. The proper use of alcohol is not sinful. The *misuse* of alcohol is sinful. And the misuse of alcohol primarily manifests itself in overindulgence, which leads to intoxication. Alcohol is celebrated in Scripture, but it must be used in moderation.

If alcohol is treated as a gift in the Scriptures, moderate use being celebrated and excessive use being condemned, can the same be said for marijuana? Is there such a thing as responsible moderate use of marijuana? That is a critical question we will address in the next chapter. But first, we have to determine why the Bible condemns intoxication.

The Bible: Intoxication Is Wrong

The primary way that the Scriptures speak to intoxication is alcohol-induced drunkenness. Some may protest that there is a significant difference between getting high on marijuana and getting drunk on alcohol. No doubt there are differences, and I do not want to discount them.

But as we look at what the Bible has to say about drunkenness, I think we will find that there are necessary implications for marijuana.

Being high on pot and drunk on alcohol both impair cognitive abilities, judgment, and physical capacities. Those are the exact reasons the Bible roundly and repeatedly forbids drunkenness.

The narratives of Scripture record the drunkenness of people, and almost without exception the implications are negative. Noah famously planted a vineyard, harvested some grapes, made wine, "became drunk, and uncovered himself inside his tent" (Gen. 9:21). We really don't know what "uncovered himself" means, but there is no chance that it was a good thing; after all, lots of trouble ensued. Lot's daughters got their father drunk so they could sleep with him (Gen. 19:30–38). Nabal, the pathetic husband of Abigail, whose name means "stupid," dangerously treated David with contempt, then topped off his day by holding a feast "fit for a king," getting "very drunk" (1 Sam. 25:36). Only after he sobered up could his wife confront him with his foolishness. It was common practice for the kings and conspirators in the hot mess that was Israelite politics to get drunk and engage in unrighteous acts (e.g., 1 Kings 16:9; 20:16). Jesus used drunkenness as a negative example in teaching (Luke 12:45). The crowds gathered at Pentecost that heard the strange speech coming from the mouths of the Spirit-anointed disciples were not complimenting them when they "sneered and said, 'They're drunk on new wine'" (Acts 2:13). Finally, Paul rebuked the Corinthian church for getting drunk during the Lord's Supper (1 Cor. 11:21).

There are also straightforward prohibitions on getting drunk. Mosaic law describes the criminally disobedient son as "a glutton and a drunkard" (Deut. 21:20). Paul commanded the Ephesian believers, "Don't get drunk with wine, which leads to reckless living, but be filled by the Spirit" (Eph. 5:18), and both Paul and Peter list drunkenness among a list of rather heinous sins (Rom. 13:13; 1 Cor. 5:11; Gal. 5:19–21; and 1 Pet. 4:3).

The Bible is clear: drunkenness, which is intoxication, is sinful.

The Bible: But Why Is Intoxication Wrong?

It is a kindness of the Lord that he does not merely forbid drunkenness in a "because I said so" manner. He could have done that. As our Creator and God, he certainly has that right. Instead, he tells us why he prohibits drunkenness, and it is here that the links between intoxication by alcohol and by marijuana can be found.

Consider Proverbs 23:29–35:

> Who has woe? Who has sorrow?
> Who has conflicts? Who has complaints?
> Who has wounds for no reason?
> Who has red eyes?
> Those who linger over wine;
> those who go looking for mixed wine.
> Don't gaze at wine because it is red,
> because it gleams in the cup
> and goes down smoothly.
> In the end it bites like a snake
> and stings like a viper.
> Your eyes will see strange things,
> and you will say absurd things.
> You'll be like someone sleeping out at sea
> or lying down on the top of a ship's mast.
> "They struck me, but I feel no pain!
> They beat me, but I didn't know it!
> When will I wake up?
> I'll look for another drink."

Here the plight of the addict is vividly described. Woe, sorrow, conflicts, complaints, wounds, red eyes—these are what is in store for those who "linger over wine." The intoxicating effects are evident as well—seeing things, saying absurd things. The drunkard is even beaten but is apparently unaware. So strong are the yearnings that even after all this, the drunkard goes looking for another drink.

God condemns drunkenness because it impairs physical control. It causes even priests and prophets to stagger and stumble (Isa. 28:7). Sometimes that lack of physical control is degrading: "Indeed, all their tables are covered with vomit; there is no place without a stench" (v. 8).

Drunkenness impairs cognitive abilities. It causes confusion (v. 7). The drunkard sees things and says absurd things (Prov. 23:33). The foolishness caused by drunkenness manifests itself in poor financial decisions (Prov. 21:17; 23:21).

Drunkenness impairs judgment. Drunkenness causes "muddled . . . visions" and people to "stumble in their judgments" (Isa. 28:7). Beer and wine create brawlers and mockers (Prov. 20:1). Kings and rulers who are preoccupied with beer and wine will "forget what is decreed," and when they do that, they will "pervert justice for all the oppressed" (Prov. 31:4–5). Even worse, those addicted to alcohol lose spiritual insight: "They do not perceive the LORD's actions, and they do not see the work of his hands" (Isa. 5:11–12).

So we see that the Scriptures give us two principles to inform our exploration of marijuana use: alcohol abuse can lead to addiction, and drunkenness is wrong because it impairs cognitive ability, judgment, and physical ability. We established in the last chapter that the same is true of marijuana: it is addictive and creates a high that impairs cognitive ability, judgment, and physical ability.

Addiction and impaired cognitive ability, physical ability, and judgment are all at odds with what is required of the follower of Jesus Christ. In contrast to addiction, Scripture places a high value on self-control. In Titus 2, Paul instructed his colleague to "proclaim things consistent with sound teaching" (v. 1). Among these "things" is the mandate that Christians are to "be self-controlled" (Titus 2:2, 5, 6). Addiction causes behaviors that are the opposite of self-controlled. Instead, the substance or behavior is exercising control over the addict.

Disciples of the Lord are to live intentionally—mind, body, and heart. Jesus Christ does not just want the spiritual aspect of the Christian's life (whatever that is). He redeemed the totality of who we are, and he therefore demands that the totality of who we are be submitted to him.

Paul taught the Christians in Rome,

> Therefore, brothers and sisters, in view of
> the mercies of God, I urge you to present

> your bodies as a living sacrifice, holy and
> pleasing to God; this is your true wor-
> ship. Do not be conformed to this age,
> but be transformed by the renewing of
> your mind, so that you may discern what
> is the good, pleasing, and perfect will of
> God. (Rom. 12:1–2)

Our bodies are to be offered to the Lord as a "living sacrifice." No doubt that language is strange to us, but it certainly means that we devote the entirety of who we are and what we do with our bodies to God because what we do with our bodies matters to God. In fact, Paul describes our bodily devotion to the Lord as "holy and pleasing to God" and "true worship." He goes on to warn against being "conformed" or squeezed into the world's mold, to adopt its way of thinking. Instead, you are to "be transformed by the renewing of your mind."

The path to such renewing is laid out by Paul in the previous eleven chapters of his letter to the Roman Christians. It includes such things as Spirit circumcision of the heart (Rom. 2), justification and redemption in Christ (Rom. 3), belief in the promises of God (Rom. 4–5), consciously offering ourselves to God rather than to sin (Rom. 6), and walking with the Spirit (Rom. 8). But notice the purpose of a renewed mind: "So that you may discern what is the good, pleasing, and perfect will of God" (Rom. 12:2). Discernment, a necessary component of moral judgment, is vital to the Christian life because it enables the Christian to live in a manner that pleases the Lord. Remember, the Bible does not tell us exactly what to do in every possible circumstance. Therefore, it takes discernment to know the right thing to do and the right way to do it.

The two verses at the beginning of Romans 12 speak directly to the issues of addiction and impaired physical ability, cognitive ability, and judgment. The opposite of the Romans 12, renewed-mind Christian is the unwise doubter of James 1. That person is "double-minded and unstable in all his ways" (v. 8). Such a person "should not expect to receive anything from the Lord" (v. 7).

The Christian life is to be lived intentionally, with no divided loyalties and no double-mindedness. It takes the totality of who we are—body, mind, and heart—to follow Jesus in a way that honors him. In the next chapter we will take a deeper look, asking questions the follower of Christ should consider when debating whether to use recreational marijuana.

CHAPTER 5

Discipleship and Marijuana

In doing some research for my presentations on this topic, I visited one of the seemingly ubiquitous marijuana dispensaries near my house. The staff at this shop were extremely patient and helpful, answering many of my questions by pulling out large visual aids with charts and graphics, showing me the different THC products and how they worked. At one point, I asked, rather embarrassingly, if there was any reason to smoke pot recreationally other than to get high. The clerk looked at me like I was an imbecile and laughed, "Why else would anybody smoke pot?"

Good question.

In speaking to marijuana users, there are two primary reasons given for *recreational* marijuana use: (1) to enjoy the pleasure marijuana brings, and (2) to escape, if only for a moment, the troubles that surround.[1] Both of those reasons require a level of mind alteration to achieve.

Perhaps you are a Christian who is unconvinced by my arguments and questions up to this point. The Scriptures are clear that intoxication is sinful, so to use marijuana for the purpose of getting high is forbidden. But maybe you advocate its use for other reasons, such as clarity of thought, or even as an aid to an enhanced relationship with God. In this chapter I want to address five questions every Christian should consider before choosing to use marijuana. By thinking through these questions, I believe Christians can reach clarity regarding the use of marijuana. I begin with the same basic question I asked the dispensary clerk.

Is There Any Reason to Smoke Pot Recreationally Other Than to Get High?

We have established that drunkenness is explicitly forbidden in the Bible. I argued that the reasons the Bible gives for prohibiting drunkenness—namely, impaired physical

---

[1] Other reasons given include relaxation, enhanced creativity, and enhanced spirituality. I will address each of these in due course.

abilities, impaired cognitive abilities, and impaired judgment—are all applicable to the marijuana high.

I also argued that alcohol is a gift from God to be enjoyed in moderation. Can the same be said for marijuana? Generally speaking, it is difficult to give an affirmative response.

In contrast to alcohol, which is digested, marijuana is most often consumed through smoking or vaping and only secondarily through digestion of edibles. Absorption rates into the bloodstream via the lungs through smoke or vapor are so high that cannabis use is typically not coupled with adjectives like *mild*, *moderate*, or *innocuous*.

People enjoy the aroma and flavor of alcohol. I rarely hear testimonies of the ambrosia-like odors of cannabis. Though there are cannabis-scented candles, most describe the smell of pot as fetid, not fragrant.

Some people consume alcohol because of its relaxing effects. Marijuana certainly has a relaxing effect on many users, but can that effect be achieved without intoxication? Some advocates argue for microdosing, which allows one to get a small amount of THC without risking intoxication.[2] But those uses are driven by medical concerns

---

[2] See, for example, Abbie Rosner, "How to Get the Health Benefits of Cannabis without Getting High," *Next Avenue*, April

(e.g., chronic pain, anxiety, sleeplessness), not recreational applications.

Though the line between recreational use and medical use of marijuana is increasingly blurry, I think recreational and medical marijuana are two different things. I will treat medical marijuana in the next chapter.

To conclude, then, it seems there is no good or logically consistent reason to smoke pot *recreationally* other than to get high.

Can You Be "Sober-Minded" While Using Marijuana?

"Therefore, with your minds ready for action, be sober-minded and set your hope completely on the grace to be brought to you at the revelation of Jesus Christ" (1 Pet. 1:13).

In Peter's first letter, after acknowledging that his readers were being persecuted for their faith, he explained that the purpose of their trials was to purify their faith so that Christ might be glorified (1 Pet. 1:6–9). But as they underwent those trials, Peter instructed that Christians must be "sober-minded" if they are to endure faithfully (1 Pet. 1:13). He called for Christians to be sober-minded

10, 2019, https://www.nextavenue.org/health-benefits-cannabis-without-getting-high.

two more times in the same short letter (1 Pet. 4:7; 5:8). Paul used the same word (*nēphō*) three times in his letters, this time translated "self-controlled"—twice to the Thessalonians that they might be ready when Christ returned (1 Thess. 5:6, 8) and once to Timothy as he exhorted the young pastor to steadfastly fulfill his ministry responsibilities (2 Tim. 4:5).

Being sober-minded is the opposite of being intoxicated. It has to do with being alert and wakeful, not drowsy. Peter's and Paul's calls for sober-mindedness are calls for the Christian to be watchful, ready for whatever weapons the enemy might wield against the believer. So a command to be sober-minded is far more than just a prohibition on intoxication, *but it is not less.*

You cannot be sober-minded if you are high. Peter was concerned that a failure to be sober-minded would result in hopes not fully resting on the grace of Christ. The implication is that having a mind that is addled by THC will get in the way of grace.

Will THC Diminish My Ability to Honor Christ in My Thinking?

The apostle Paul taught that disciples of Christ "do not wage war according to the flesh" (2 Cor. 10:3). Rather, the Christian arsenal is not of this world. Paul elaborated,

> Since the weapons of our warfare are not of the flesh, but are powerful through God for the demolition of strongholds. We demolish arguments and every proud thing that is raised up against the knowledge of God, and we take every thought captive to obey Christ. (2 Cor. 10:4–5)

Paul was candid throughout 2 Corinthians that the human mind is the primary locale of spiritual warfare. Christians are not to be "ignorant of [Satan's] schemes" (2 Cor. 2:11). Satan has "blinded the minds of the unbelievers to keep them from seeing the light of the gospel of the glory of Christ" (2 Cor. 4:4). Paul later warned that Satan attempts to deceive believers just as he did Eve in the garden (2 Cor. 11:3). Therefore, Paul exhorted the Corinthian believers to "demolish arguments" (2 Cor. 10:4) against the truth and knowledge of God and to bring everybody's thoughts under the lordship of Christ.

Furthermore, the Christian is to be ready to proclaim the truth at all times, what Paul called "in season and out of season" (2 Tim. 4:2). Shifting into preacher autopilot mode, when given the opportunity, is not what Paul is getting at. No, the Christian must be able to discern any situation at hand and provide the appropriate truth from God's Word at the appropriate time. That requires the Christian to listen to the Spirit while analyzing the situation. Peter uses the same logic when he instructs, "In your hearts regard Christ the Lord as holy, ready at any time to give a defense to anyone who asks you for a reason for the hope that is in you" (1 Pet. 3:15).

Is it possible to do that if your brain is under the influence of THC? At my presentations, I have talked to confessing Christians who are adamant that they think more clearly when using marijuana. I have no wish to argue with someone's experience because I cannot do so. But remember, THC decreases firing in the hippocampus, the part of the brain that regulates learning and the assimilation of new information. It may be true that a person thinks more clearly when he or she is high; even if it is true, this would not be a solution but a revelation that the person's mind is overly clouded, distracted, or busy when not high. If this is the case, there are much more effective and less harmful techniques to combat mental cloudiness.

The ability to "demolish arguments and every proud thing that is raised up against the knowledge of God" and to "take every thought captive to obey Christ" (2 Cor. 10:4–5) is impaired when the Christian's mind is under the influence of THC.

Following Christ requires clear-minded intentionality and perspective. We are asked to examine ourselves to see if we are in the faith (2 Cor. 13:5). We are to "approve the things that are superior" so that we might be "pure and blameless in the day of Christ" (Phil. 1:10). Is the introduction of a mind-altering chemical that demonstrably distorts thinking going to aid the Christian in such discernment and examination? Gaining perspective and clarity while battling the world, the flesh, and the devil is problematic enough. Why add to the difficulty by introducing a psychoactive drug into the mix?

> Gaining perspective and clarity while battling the world, the flesh, and the devil is problematic enough. Why add to the difficulty by introducing a psychoactive drug into the mix?

Will THC Diminish My Ability to Honor Christ in My Actions?

Peter's command to be sober minded in 1 Peter 1:13 was given so that the Christian's mind might be "ready for action." John instructed that love was to be performed "in action and in truth" (1 John 3:18). Paul highlights the importance of intentional discipline and action when he compared the Christian life to that of the soldier, the athlete, and the farmer.

> Share in suffering as a good soldier of Christ Jesus. No one serving as a soldier gets entangled in the concerns of civilian life; he seeks to please the commanding officer. Also, if anyone competes as an athlete, he is not crowned unless he competes according to the rules. The hardworking farmer ought to be the first to get a share of the crops. (2 Tim. 2:3–6)

The disciple of Christ is to be like a soldier in his single-minded devotion and obedience to Christ. The Christian, like the athlete, is charged to compete and to do so in compliance with the rules. And the farmer who gets a share in the crops is described as hardworking. These three images have everything to do with engagement, intentionality, and a work ethic. Such things are to characterize the Christian.

Are those attributes often correlated with marijuana use? Consider the negative impact of marijuana on ambition and motivation (summarized in chapter 2), and ask whether marijuana will aid or hinder your discipleship and ability to be faithful to all the Lord calls you to do. Pastor Jeff Lacine helpfully warns, "There is a reason that marijuana has long been associated with the couch, a bag of chips, and a television remote. . . . Regular marijuana use causes disengagement, dulling individuals into a long-term, slow, and subtle numbness. If you ask almost anyone who has formerly used cannabis on a regular basis, he will speak about this phenomenon."[3]

Lacine's warning is apt. The Christian life is to be lived with intentionality. People do not grow in Christlikeness through passivity. Sanctification is achieved, by God's grace, by actively refusing to offer yourself to sin and by offering all parts of yourself to God to be used by him (Rom. 6:12–13).

---

[3] Jeff Lacine, "Marijuana to the Glory of God?," desiringGod, January 7, 2017, https://www.desiringgod.org/articles/marijuana-to-the-glory-of-god.

It has been clinically demonstrated that THC does not engender greater personal ambition but leads to inaction. Discipling others, on the other hand, requires a plan and intentional engagement. Evangelism requires awareness of those around you and a determination to share the gospel. The spiritual disciplines of prayer, Scripture reading, meditation, and fasting are rightly named "disciplines" because they require a plan and the fortitude to carve out the time to pursue the Lord. Will any of these vital activities be elevated by THC?

Will THC Enhance My Ability to Commune with God?

A growing number of people swear by the spiritual powers of marijuana. California is home to a number of "cannabis churches," places of worship where cannabis is treated as a sacrament.[4] Many of the so-called cannabis churches are far from orthodox, a syncretistic blend of Christianity, Judaism, Rastafarianism, and Buddhism. But some more mainstream and evangelical Christian leaders are calling for a reevaluation of the typical negative

---

[4] See Arit John, "Inside the War for California's Cannabis Churches," *The New York Times*, November 23, 2019, https://www.nytimes.com/2019/11/23/style/weed-church-california.html.

Christian response to marijuana.[5] For most of these, the reasons are medical. But some Christians are eager to explore the supposed spiritual benefits of marijuana.

An entheogen is a chemical substance with psychoactive effects that is ingested to alter consciousness for spiritual purposes. Cannabis is touted by some Christians for its ability to remove the veil of illusion, to illuminate you from within, and to quiet the noise. In this space, they say, you can connect to yourself and to God. Collette Patricia, a member of the Christian Cannabis team, an organization started by XXXChurch founding pastor Craig Gross, writes, "When used with intention and respect, cannabis is spiritual. It can show you a side of yourself that you've never seen before. A side of you that is divine."[6] (Remember what I said about confusing the Creator-creature distinction in chapter 3?)

In the websites I visited for "cannabis churches," I found far more space committed to marijuana distribution

---

[5] Jonathan Merritt, "The Christian Case for Marijuana," *The New York Times*, June 20, 2019, sec. Opinion, https://www nytimes.com/2019/06/20/opinion/legalization-medical-marijuana -christianity.html.

[6] Collette Patricia, *Cannabis Is Spiritual* (Spiritual Plants, 2019). Accessed at cannabisisspiritual.com.

than sound doctrine or an affirmation of the gospel.[7] And the goals of removing the veil of illusion and quieting the noise so as to find God within has more to do with new age mysticism than "the faith that was delivered to the saints once for all" (Jude 3). Even the churches that claim to be Christian offer meditations that have far more in common with Buddhism than Christianity. A typical example would find a meditation leader, in the lotus position, inviting the participants to consume their marijuana and then guiding them through relaxation and centering techniques.[8] Those who watch online are treated to a moving kaleidoscope filling the screen. The International Church of Cannabis, whose chapel walls are painted with a cacophony of psychedelic colors and patterns more reminiscent of Scooby-Doo's Mystery Machine than the Sistine Chapel, offers an hourly "Guided Meditation and Laser Light Experience."[9]

---

[7] "Cannabis churches" are in an intense battle with state governments, which see them as little more than unlicensed marijuana distribution centers. The "cannabis churches" have named cannabis as a sacrament and have sought protection under the Religious Freedom Restoration Act of 1993. John, "Inside the War for California's Cannabis Churches."

[8] For an example, go to cannabisisspiritual.com/meditation.

[9] The International Church of Cannabis makes no claims to be Christian, though Christians are welcome. Instead, members of the church identify as "elevationists" who have "no divine law,

Advocates claim that marijuana is an aid to meditation. That may be true, but it depends on the kind of meditation being practiced. Eastern meditation associated with enlightenment and becoming one with the universe, by repeating a mantra, may be aided by psychoactive drugs like marijuana. But the meditation prescribed in the Bible does not resemble such practices.

Joshua was told, "This book of instruction must not depart from your mouth; you are to meditate on it day and night so that you may carefully observe everything written in it" (Josh. 1:8). The psalmist describes the blessed as those whose "delight is in the LORD's instruction" and who "meditates on it day and night" (Ps. 1:2). The Hebrew word translated "meditate" is *hagah*, and it literally means "to mutter over." Far from emptying our minds, biblical meditation is about filling our minds with the Word of God and thinking about it so intensely that we find ourselves talking out loud. Again, will mind-altering drugs enable more faithful reflection on the promises and character of God as recorded in Holy Scripture?

Consider the priority the Scriptures place on seeing God. The psalms use the metaphor of "seeing the Lord"

no unquestionable doctrine, and no authoritarian structure." See www.elevationists.org.

for knowing God. Seeing the Lord is the fulfillment of the ultimate hope of his people. The righteous "will see" the face of the Lord (Ps. 11:7). People are invited to "taste and see that the LORD is good" (Ps. 34:8). When people "see and fear" the Lord, they will trust in him (Ps. 40:3). Jesus and the New Testament authors also used the metaphor of seeing God to describe the essence of the Christian walk and hope. Jesus announced that the pure in heart would see God (Matt 5:8). The author of Hebrews calls people to pursue peace and holiness, because without them, "no one will see the Lord" (Heb. 12:14). John wrote, "Dear friends, we are God's children now, and what we will be has not yet been revealed. We know that when he appears, we will be like him because we will see him as he is" (1 John 3:2). Paul famously described the Christian's current situation and future hope with the sight metaphor:

> For we know in part, and we prophesy
> in part, but when the perfect comes, the
> partial will come to an end. When I was a
> child, I spoke like a child, I thought like
> a child, I reasoned like a child. When I
> became a man, I put aside childish things.
> For now we see only a reflection as in a
> mirror, but then face to face. Now I know

in part, but then I will know fully, as I am
fully known. (1 Cor. 13:9–12)

Paul taught that we will know fully only when the "perfect comes." Most understand the "perfect" to be the return of Christ at the consummation of this age. Few would argue that the "perfect" is a cannabinoid or some other entheogen.

The problem of our spiritual blindness is only overcome through grace. Only God is able to "give the light of the knowledge of God's glory in the face of Jesus Christ" (2 Cor. 4:6). Lack of holiness clouds our ability to see God. The human predicament is one of spiritual blindness and death caused by rebellion and sin. It is *not* the result of not having the right psychoactive chemical introduced to our brains.

The idea that marijuana could unlock portals to a newer and better relationship with the Lord is sub-Christian and makes a mockery of grace and of our true predicament.

Far from affirming entheogens, Scripture warns against mind-altering drugs. We discussed Ephesians 5:18 earlier, but it bears repeating

Far from enabling better sight and vision of God, marijuana distorts reality and clouds moral judgment.

here. Paul contrasts getting "drunk with wine" (forbidden) and being "filled by the Spirit" (commanded). There is no place for intoxication in a faithful life before God. To suggest that drugs are a valuable aid to worship and piety is to ignore the entirety of Scripture's teachings on the role of the mind and correct thinking in discipleship. Far from enabling better sight and vision of God, marijuana distorts reality and clouds moral judgment. In order to assert a biblical category for entheogens, you have to insert it into the Scriptures first. Entheogens just aren't there.

Navigating Gray Areas

In a previous chapter, I mentioned that there is a category of decisions we daily make with no clear moral implications. These indifferent matters, or *adiaphora*, are not always easy to navigate, and the Bible provides no inspired exhaustive list of them. Paul famously wrote to the Corinthian church about eating meat that had been sacrificed to idols. In 1 Corinthians 10, Paul argued that if you were participating in an idolatrous ceremony where the meat is served, then this is not an indifferent matter—it is clearly sin. But in 1 Corinthians 8, Paul taught that meat bought in the marketplace was just meat, even if it had been earlier sacrificed to an idol. Feel free to eat that meat with a clear conscience.

Unless . . .

If, by eating the meat sacrificed to an idol, the Corinthian Christian caused a brother or sister in Christ to sin, then what was formerly permitted was then forbidden. Let me say that again: if an action that in and of itself is not forbidden is a stumbling block to other Christians, then it becomes a sin. Sometimes an activity is okay and other times it's not, depending on who is watching.

The principle is that Paul refused to exercise a freedom if in doing so he would cause a fellow Christian to sin. "Therefore, if food causes my brother or sister to fall, I will never again eat meat, so that I won't cause my brother or sister to fall" (1 Cor. 8:13).

Gray areas are tricky because what might be right in one instance becomes wrong in the next. So, how do we navigate such things?

Perhaps some of you are persuaded that there is nothing wrong with recreational marijuana as long as you do not get intoxicated. I haven't convinced you, and you view such recreational marijuana use a gray area. If so, I have found the following list of questions to be helpful in making decisions about indifferent matters in my own life.[10] I explain each of the questions with specific application to marijuana, but the questions are applicable to any morally indifferent activity.

    1. *Am I fully persuaded that this activity is right?* (Rom. 14:14, 22–23). Is smoking pot truly an indifferent matter? Have you considered all of the risks? Have you considered the biblical prohibition on intoxication and believe that you can partake of marijuana without violating those prohibitions? Remember, whatever is not done in faith is sin. If you are not sure whether smoking marijuana is right and permissible, then refrain until such time as you are fully persuaded.

    2. *Can I practice the activity as "for the Lord"?* (Rom 14:6–8). God is the giver of all good things. Can you smoke pot or consume an edible and then thank

---

[10] I was given most of these questions by Gregg Allison in a class on pastoral ethics that I took during my MDiv studies at Western Seminary, and I have been using them ever since.

the Lord for the good gift of marijuana he just gave you?

3. *Can I engage in the activity without being a stumbling block to my brothers and sisters in Christ?* (Rom. 14:13, 15, 20–21). If your pot smoking is going to lead a brother or sister to violate their conscience by following your example, then you should refrain. Are others going to be encouraged to use marijuana who will not be able to use it without sinning, because they see or know that you are doing so? Even if you managed to practice "micro-dosing" and used pot without achieving a high, can you be assured the people you influence would do the same?

4. *Does the activity promote righteousness, peace, and joy?* (Rom 14:17, 19a). Is your pot smoking going to promote the characteristics of the kingdom of God? Many Christians today are so anxious to exercise their freedom in Christ that they forget the example of their Lord who emptied himself

and gave up his life (Phil. 2:6–8) for the sake of the kingdom of God. Flaunting your liberty in Christ by smoking pot to demonstrate your freedom to others is a poor motivation and will be more divisive than peace and righteousness promoting.

5. *Does the activity edify others?* (Rom. 14:19b). Christians should be all about building others up. If your marijuana use is going to bring harm to another, then you should refrain. What about your younger brother or sister? The children in your youth group, or the ones who call you "Mom" or "Dad"? Will this edify them?

6. *Is this practice profitable?* (1 Cor. 6:12a). Paul is clear that even if "all" things are permissible, not all things are beneficial. He therefore establishes a criterion that is more limiting because you ought to do only those things that are profitable. His reasoning gives us a glimpse into his intensity. Like all humans, he had a finite

amount of time and energy, and he did not want to waste them on activities that were not profitable. So, even if you have the liberty to consume marijuana, is it profitable?

7. *Does this activity enslave me?* (1 Cor. 6:12b). Paul's second criterion in 1 Corinthians 6 is that he did not want to do anything that might enslave him. This question is especially crucial for the topic of marijuana. Is there potential for marijuana use to enslave you? Can you become addicted? Will your desire for pot be so great that you make unwise or sinful decisions to fulfill that need? Will your family see a difference in your personality or desires and regret your enslavement?

8. *Does this activity bring glory to God?* (1 Cor. 10:31). As disciples of Christ, we are to do all things for the glory of God. So the question is, Will God be glorified through your pot consumption?

9. *Is the Holy Spirit guiding me into this activity?* (Gal. 5:16–18; Rom. 8). The Holy Spirit is fully God, so if the Holy Spirit is guiding you into an activity, you absolutely have full divine approval for engaging in it. The question is one of discernment. How might you know that the Spirit is guiding you to smoke marijuana? You might have noticed that many of the questions are interrelated. For example, it would be difficult to defend the claim that the Holy Spirit was guiding you to smoke pot if you did not believe it was profitable, edifying, or promoted the things of the kingdom.

Many Christians today are so anxious to exercise their freedom in Christ that they forget the example of their Lord who emptied himself and gave up his life.

These questions might seem restrictive. You might be thinking that if you have to get the right answers to all those questions before you do anything, it would be better to just stay in bed! First, "staying in bed" is itself an activity, and doing so to avoid sin will probably not pass the test of those questions. Second, and far more importantly, the questions do not restrict good activities done for good reasons. But they will restrict bad activities or good activities done for the wrong reasons.

I just got back from playing disc golf with my boys. It was fun, recreating, edifying, peace promoting, and God glorifying. That activity at that time passed every one of the tests. I ate one of my daughter's cupcakes after lunch and was grateful to God and her for that tasty treat. What's more, I didn't have to take the time to run through the question checklist. It was the right thing to do, and I am grateful to be able to do such things. Of course, if I start neglecting my family or other responsibilities in my hopeless quest to be a disc golf professional, or if I am on my seventh cupcake of the day, the answers to the questions would be different.

Even with those examples, you still might feel that following Christ should not be that hard. Doesn't he want you to have fun? What's the problem with getting high now and then?

I have been a follower of Jesus Christ for almost all of my life. My testimony is that Christ wants to bring you joy (John 16:24).

And it's going to be hard.

Sometimes you will have to deny your desires. But the path on which Jesus leads you is a path to eternal life. He came that our joy might be complete (John 16:24), that we would be able to rejoice in all our circumstances, even in our trials (1 Pet. 4:13). I can honestly say that I have never regretted any decision I have made to obey Jesus, even though those choices were often difficult.

Jesus likened following him with taking up a cross and dying to self (Luke 9:23). Jesus is not a bait-and-switch salesman. He never promised you that following him would be easy or fun all the time. Far from it. But he did promise that following him would be worth it.

CHAPTER 6

How Does Medical Marijuana Work?

Marijuana cured my father of cancer!"

The woman who waited until the end of my presentation to share her experience with me was like many who have spoken to me after hearing me teach on recreational and medical marijuana. In her case, she explained that her father's diagnosis was severe, the prognosis was most likely terminal, and that nothing had worked until he tried medical marijuana. As the conversation continued, her friend added that the woman's father had continued to get other, conventional treatment. But the daughter sincerely believed the marijuana was instrumental in her father's current good health. I could multiply examples like this.

But what can be said, with confidence, about the efficacy of medical marijuana? Do research and science support the claims of the marijuana industry regarding the many medical conditions cannabis can treat?

All my early presentations were on the recreational use of marijuana. What soon became evident was that many of the most perplexing questions for Christians surrounded "medical marijuana." I learned to be specific in my presentations that I was talking about recreational marijuana and later added a separate presentation on medical marijuana. Here is what I found.

Some doctors, not most, are now recommending marijuana to patients. I say "recommend" because marijuana cannot be prescribed per se. A "prescription" can mean at least a couple of things. In the broad sense, a prescription can be any regimen a doctor recommends, such as taking daily walks, lowering salt intake, or avoiding peanuts. In that sense a physician can prescribe marijuana joints or edibles.

The more common use of the word *prescription* refers to a written order for a medication at a specific dose, which can be filled at a medical pharmacy. I will be using that more narrow sense of prescription in the remainder of this book.

Dosage from a joint or edible is not possible to control given the different THC percentages and idiosyncratic responses to pot. It's not like a doctor can control the dose by saying, "Smoke two joints and call me in the morning." And marijuana is still a Schedule 1 drug. According to the United States Drug Enforcement Agency (DEA), Schedule 1 drugs have "*no currently accepted medical use in the United States,* a lack of accepted safety for use under medical supervision, and a high potential for abuse."[1] Nevertheless, the use of marijuana for medical purposes is legal in thirty-three states (and Washington, DC) in America. When a patient is suffering from nausea, lack of appetite, or pain, it is becoming more and more common for a doctor to suggest that a patient consider trying marijuana.

Some Christians readily accept the recommendation. A few Christians have been self-medicating with marijuana for a number of years to fight nausea, pain, lack of appetite, neuropathy, anxiety, depression, and a number of other maladies. But other Christians are not so sure. There is a stigma attached to smoking marijuana, probably because it

---

[1] U.S. Department of Justice, Drug Enforcement Administration, "Controlled Substance Schedules," https://www.deadiversion.usdoj .gov/schedules/index.html.

has been illegal for so long, but also because Christians are concerned about its mind-altering effects.

The purpose of this chapter is to explore the efficacy of medical marijuana. We will find that components of the cannabis plant have a proven medical benefit, and there are approved drugs from those components. But the claims of medical marijuana advocates far outpace the hard evidence. In order for Christians to make good decisions about whether to use marijuana for medical purposes, there must be clarity on what the drug does not do, what it may do, and what it has been proven to do.

> **The claims of medical marijuana advocates far outpace the hard evidence.**

What Exactly Is Medical Marijuana?

Medical marijuana is just marijuana used for medical purposes. The medicinal properties of marijuana have been lauded for more than five thousand years around the world. Medical marijuana is the same plant, often bought from the same batch at the same dispensary, as recreational marijuana.

In fact, the use of the term *medical marijuana* is somewhat controversial since the U.S. Food and Drug

Administration (FDA) has not recognized or approved the marijuana plant as medicine. So, at this stage, marijuana, even if it is called "medical marijuana," is not medicine per se. Parts of the marijuana plant *have* become medicine, and other parts *may* become medicine.

An illustration will be helpful. Historically, the drug quinine has been used to treat malaria.[2] Quinine is developed from the bark of the cinchona tree. Doctors would not treat malaria by prescribing cinchona tree bark to their patients. Rather, they would prescribe specific doses of the drug developed from the tree bark. In the same way, drugs developed from components of the marijuana plant can be isolated and prescribed. Dosage from those drugs can be controlled. Marijuana itself is more problematic from a pharmaceutical standpoint. As psychiatrists Dr. Herbert Kleber and Dr. Robert DuPont opine, "Medical marijuana laws challenge physicians to recommend use of a Schedule 1 illegal drug of abuse with no scientific approval, dosage control, or quality control."[3]

---

[2] I heard this illustration from Dr. Greg Bledsoe on Heathcott Associates, *No Dope_Complete*, 2016, https://vimeo.com/184363767.

[3] Herbert D. Kleber, and Robert L. DuPont, "Physicians and Medical Marijuana," *American Journal of Psychiatry* 169:6 (June 2012): 564–68.

How Does Medical Marijuana Work?

Since medical marijuana is the same plant as recreational marijuana, the science behind medical marijuana is the same. Medical marijuana affects the body in the same ways as recreational marijuana. So, everything that was said in chapter 1, "What Is Marijuana and How Does It Work?," for recreational marijuana, applies to medical marijuana. There is the same risk of addiction, the same risk to heart and lungs, the same risks to teenage brain development, and the same potential for mental health issues.

What Are the Medical Uses of Marijuana?

The cannabis plant is complex, with many different components. Because marijuana is a Schedule 1 drug, no studies have been done on the long-term use of those components for medicinal purposes. It is established scientifically that THC (a psychoactive cannabinoid) increases appetite and reduces nausea. To date, the FDA has approved two THC medicines in pill form (dronabinol and nabilone) for those purposes. These medicines are of benefit for those struggling with the side effects of chemotherapy who fail to respond to conventional anti-emetic (anti-vomiting) medicines.

To be clear, when a doctor prescribes one of these medications, she is not prescribing marijuana. Patients would pick up the medication at a pharmacy. You cannot buy marijuana (even if used for medical purposes) at a pharmacy.

Interestingly, advocates for medical marijuana often mention a range of medical illnesses for which marijuana may be effective: cancer, glaucoma, HIV, hepatitis C, ALS, Crohn's disease, Parkinson's disease, multiple sclerosis, etc. The problem is that there is little scientific support for these claims. At best the evidence is weak. For most it is nonexistent. In the case of glaucoma, for example, the negative side effects of marijuana use outweigh the potential benefits, and the Glaucoma Research Foundation does not recommend the use of cannabinoids for treatment of glaucoma.[4]

There is much anecdotal evidence that THC decreases pain, inflammation, and muscle control problems. There have been a number of studies looking at the effectiveness

---

[4] Henry D. Jampel, "Should You Be Smoking Marijuana to Treat Your Glaucoma?" *Glaucoma Research Foundation*, October 29, 2017, https://www.glaucoma.org/treatment/should-you-be-smoking -marijuana-to-treat-your-glaucoma-1.php.

of cannabinoids at treating chronic pain, but the results are inconclusive. About half of the studies show hopeful signs, while the other half show no significant benefit at all. It is thought that THC may help users cope with pain, but there is inconclusive evidence that it diminishes pain intensity.

Unfortunately, taking medical marijuana to cope with pain puts one in the realm of greatest abuse. As of 2020, the U.S. FDA had not approved any cannabinoids for pain relief. THC works as an intoxicant first and as a pain reliever second. It is not a strong enough painkiller for those who would ordinarily require an opiate to control acute pain.

The studies for the control of spasticity in patients with multiple sclerosis is much the same as for chronic pain relief. The results of testing are inconclusive, with about half of scientific studies showing hopeful results and the other half demonstrating no statistically significant benefit at all. To date the FDA has not approved any cannabinoids for treatment of spasticity.

THC has been lauded for its potential to improve motor symptoms for Parkinson's disease, but unfortunately there is no evidence to support the claims. Studies have not been able to demonstrate any beneficial impact for those with Parkinson's.[5]

Many people self-medicate with marijuana products to treat their anxiety. Anecdotal evidence abounds for the benefits of marijuana on anxiety; the "mellowing" effects of marijuana are well-known. Dr. Robin Murray of King's College London has noted that "frequent cannabis users consistently have a high prevalence of anxiety disorders and patients with anxiety disorders have relatively high rates of cannabis use."[6] But research shows that in some individuals marijuana use can lead to increased anxiety and depression. Dr. Kevin Hill, professor of psychiatry and an addiction consultant, explains that marijuana can cause anxiety in two ways: "First, it can worsen generalized feelings of anxiety, and it can cause panic attacks."[7]

---

[5] "Medical Marijuana" (Parkinson's Foundation), accessed October 18, 2020, https://www.parkinson.org/Understanding-Parkinsons/Treatment/Medical-Marijuana.

[6] Robin M. Murray et al, "Cannabis, the Mind and Society: The Hash Realities," *Nature Reviews Neuroscience* vol. 8, 11 (2007): 885–95, doi:10.1038/nrn2253.

[7] Kevin P. Hill, *Marijuana: The Unbiased Truth about the World's Most Popular Weed* (Center City, MN: Hazelden Publishing, 2015), 44. Hill claims that almost three out of every four marijuana users (72%) also have a psychiatric problem like anxiety or depression. Ibid., 48. Murray, "Cannabis, the Mind and Society,"

However, the evidence is inconclusive whether marijuana use increases the risk of developing long-lasting anxiety disorders.[8]

It has been argued that marijuana is a good alternative to opioids and that marijuana use can lead to lower opioid addiction mortality rates. That has been demonstrated not to be the case. In fact, the trend was discovered to work in the opposite direction.[9] Deaths due to opioid overdose actually have increased in states that have legalized medical marijuana.

Despite the claims advanced by advocates for medical marijuana, the medical evidence, at this point, does not indicate significant demonstrable benefits. In fact, in many instances, the data moves in the opposite direction.

The following is a list of medical associations that have released position papers outlining why they do *not* support

doi:10.1038/nrn2253. R. C. Kessler, et al, "Lifetime Prevalence and Age-of-Onset Distributions of DSM-IV Disorders in the National Comorbidity Survey Replication" [published correction appears in Arch Gen Psychiatry, July 2005, 62(7):768. Kathleen R. Merikangas, *Arch Gen Psychiatry*, 62, no. 6 (2005):593–602.

[8] Murray, "Cannabis, the Mind and Society."

[9] C. L. Shover et al, "Association between Medical Cannabis Laws and Opioid Overdose Mortality Has Reversed over Time," *Proceedings of the National Academy of Sciences* 116, no. 26 (June 25, 2019): 12624–26.

the use of medical marijuana: the American Medical Association, the American Psychiatric Association, the American Academy of Addiction Psychiatry, the American Society of Addiction Medicine, and the American Academy of Child and Adolescent Psychiatry.[10] To clarify, these associations are speaking out against medical marijuana as purchased and procured at marijuana dispensaries. Their position papers do not mean the medical possibilities of marijuana have been tapped out. That is decidedly not the case. Investigation into the therapeutic power of the different isolated components of the cannabis plant has only just begun, and there is every reason to be hopeful that more helpful discoveries are on the way.

What about CBD?

CBD (cannabidiol) is a nonpsychoactive cannabinoid derived from the cannabis plant. It seems like it is sold everywhere now, from coffee and doughnut shops, to grocery stores, to, in particular, any place that sells essential oils and vitamins. Spas and resorts routinely offer CBD products as part of their services. I recently saw an advertisement for CBD pet products, suggesting that CBD has

---

[10] Hill, *Marijuana: The Unbiased Truth About the World's Most Popular Weed*, 108.

been effective in treating phobias, anxiety, glaucoma, cancer, chronic pain, and digestive issues in animals. So CBD is certainly popular and promises a lot.

Because it is not mind-altering, none of the concerns about intoxication are present. I am often asked if it is okay for a Christian to use CBD products (people are concerned that since it comes from the marijuana plant, it will be harmful or sinful). Rest assured: CBD is not psychoactive. There is no reason to feel that CBD is off-limits. If it helps you, then use it. But also be warned: it is rather expensive.

Anecdotal evidence for the benefits of CBD abounds. Scientific evidence typically lags behind personal testimony, and CBD studies are no exception here. CBD *may* be useful in reducing pain and inflammation and treating mental illness and addictions. Dr. Kevin P. Hill writes, "CBD is not psychoactive, but it does have a calming, or anti-anxiety effect, and increasing amounts of research point to CBD having antipsychotic effects as well in reducing the frequency and severity of psychotic symptoms."[11]

The impact of CBD on epileptic seizures is even more promising. In fact, the U.S. FDA has approved Epidiolex,

---

[11] Hill, *Marijuana: The Unbiased Truth about the World's Most Popular Weed*, 101.

a CBD oral solution, for the treatment of seizures associated with two rare and severe forms of epilepsy.

Interestingly, THC levels in marijuana are inversely proportional to CBD levels. Increasing the THC level will usually lower the CBD level and vice versa. Marijuana bred for a high CBD level will have a corresponding low THC level; marijuana bred for high THC levels will be low in CBD. Because growers are breeding for higher and higher THC levels, the drop in average CBD levels has been considerable. The downside of this is that the nonpsychoactive CBD may reduce the addictive effect of opioids and marijuana itself. By depleting the cannabis plant of its CBD levels to increase THC levels, growers may be robbing the plant of its protective element.

Where Do We Go from Here?

If you are convinced of the benefits of medical marijuana, this chapter might have seemed hopelessly critical. My goal is to provide you with the facts as we know them. It is not easy to wade through all the claims made by proponents and advocates. Because marijuana is a Schedule 1 drug (or was at the time of this writing), scientific studies have not been easy to perform. The result is that most of the evidence for the curative and palliative effects of marijuana is anecdotal rather than clinical and scientific.

To be certain, "anecdotal evidence" is not the same as "no evidence." Christians, of all people, should be the last to dismiss anecdotal evidence; eyewitness accounts are vital to Christianity (1 John 1:1–3), and we treasure the value of personal testimony. But when it comes to medicine, anecdotal evidence is not as reliable as scientific evidence borne out of clinical trials, which attempts to isolate as many variables as possible so that researchers can be confident they know what a drug is actually doing.

So, what is the Christian to do? Like most drugs, there are risks associated with medical marijuana use. Like opioids, THC is a mind-altering drug. Though not as addictive as opioids, THC is addictive. What questions ought the Christian to answer when considering medical marijuana? It is to that issue we turn next.

CHAPTER 7

Thinking Biblically about Medical Marijuana

In the fall of 2019, my wife, Camille, was diagnosed with cancer. Over the next nine months she underwent surgery, chemotherapy, and radiation therapy. The treatments and recovery between each were brutal.

Like every family dealing with cancer, our house became a pharmaceutical center. Drugs were taken before, during, and after the chemotherapy. The regimen of drugs was meant to bring healing to her and to counteract the side effects of the medication and treatment. Her immediate recovery from the surgery was aided by opioids, and her intense nausea during chemotherapy cycles was treated with strong psychoactive drugs. Bringing relief to her struggle was not an exact science, and it took a couple of iterations before the nausea was brought under some control. The intensity of Camille's reaction to the chemotherapy was probably worse than what is typical, and during those first three cycles of chemotherapy, I have never seen anybody as physically sick as my poor wife.

Before she began chemotherapy, my older children joked with her about the use of marijuana to control her nausea. This was particularly funny because when Camille was in the fourth grade, an overzealous Sunday school teacher asked her to make a vow to "never drink alcohol or do drugs." Camille made the vow and has kept it. During those first three cycles, the idea of using marijuana was often brought up again (by family and friends), but this time no one was joking. The doctors thankfully got her nausea under control but only with strong psychoactive drugs that kept my wife in a thick fog she absolutely hated.

Looking back on it, I am struck by a couple things. First, when she was so violently ill, she was not thinking straight at all. In terms of her engagement and critical thinking skills, there was little difference between when she was nauseated and when she was on the psychoactive drugs. Both the suffering and the drugs had a similar effect in that regard. The big difference was that she was not suffering while on the drugs.

Second, I am not sure what the difference would have been between the psychoactive drugs and any mental effects marijuana would have had on her. I don't see any morally significant difference between the relief of suffering via THC and the relief of suffering via a prescribed psychoactive drug. Both, after all, are psychoactive drugs.

In this chapter I want to address the questions that surround the use of medical marijuana by Christians. How is the Christian to wade through all the claims made by marijuana advocates? What are Christians to do if their physician recommends medical marijuana? How are Christians to react to family members, fellow church members, and friends who swear by its use?

In the last chapter, we described what medical marijuana is and what it has been proven to do. Now we can think biblically about its application. What follows is a series of biblical teachings one must consider when making the decision on whether to use marijuana for medical purposes. Much of what we look at here can be applied more broadly than just to marijuana.

A Human Is an Interrelated Combination of Material and Immaterial Parts

The first two chapters of Genesis describe the creation of Adam and Eve. Chapter 1 provides a brief summary with multiple references to the man and woman being made in the image of God and being given the delegated authority to rule on God's behalf over all that he had just made. Genesis 2 gives a more detailed account, and our attention is drawn to the care and workmanship God used to make the first man and first woman.

Since God created humans to represent him on the earth and exercise delegated authority on his behalf, it makes sense that he would equip his representatives to succeed in that task. To that end he created the man and the woman with bodies. "Then the LORD God formed the man out of the dust from the ground and breathed the breath of life into his nostrils, and the man became a living being" (Gen. 2:7). Neither the man nor the woman was created *ex nihilo*, out of nothing. The universe was created out of nothing, but God formed the man out of dirt, physical material.

But the material element was not sufficient to make the man a "living being." God had to breathe into him the "breath of life." This narrative and other biblical passages show that humans have not only a physical body but also a spiritual or immaterial element (Matt. 10:28; 1 Thess. 5:23). These two aspects, the material and the immaterial, can be separated, which is what happens at death (Gen. 3:19; Rev. 6:9–11). But death runs contrary to the design of God. The promise of Scripture is that redeemed humanity will be resurrected and embodied to live forever with God (1 Cor. 15:1–58; Rev. 20:4–6). Further, the Scriptures teach that the material and immaterial aspects are composed of many different components (like strength, mind, heart, etc.), all integrated into one united person (e.g., Luke 10:27; Deut. 6:5; Rom. 8:10; 1 Tim. 1:5).

That the human is a unified being means that what we do with the immaterial part of us impacts the material, and what we do with the material part of us impacts the immaterial. When we get hungry, we lose patience easily (think especially of young children). When we are troubled or nervous, we feel "butterflies" in our stomach. Depression can manifest itself physically, and lack of sleep can get in the way of good mental health. The material and immaterial parts of us are inextricably tied together.

> What we do with the immaterial part of us impacts the material, and what we do with the material part of us impacts the immaterial.

The story of Elijah is instructive. After his show-down with the prophets of Baal on Mount Carmel (1 Kings 18), Elijah was forced to flee for his life because of Jezebel's threats (1 Kings 19:1–3). Elijah's flight wore him out, and he was exhausted, discouraged, and despaired of his life. He wanted to die (1 Kings 19:4). The Lord sent an angel to give him his next mission, but Elijah was in no position to hear from the Lord, much less go on that mission. Two times the angel gave him food and water, and two times Elijah ate, drank, and slept (1 Kings 19:5–8). Only after Elijah was rested, nourished, and hydrated could he hear from the Lord and be in the proper place physically, emotionally, and mentally to receive and fulfill his mandate (1 Kings 19:9–18). God took care of the totality of Elijah's needs as a human, both material and immaterial.

Because humans are unified wholes composed of material and immaterial aspects, there are significant spiritual implications for what we do with our bodies. We have already discussed the body being the temple of the Lord (1 Cor. 3:16; 6:19), so we do not need to revisit that. But this doctrine teaches that God cares about our bodies, and it is sub-Christian to suggest that we can do whatever we want with our bodies without any harm to our spirit or relationship with the Lord. Thus, Christians should evaluate anything and everything before it goes into their bodies, even if it is medicine.

Suffering Is Treated Variably in Scripture

Following the glorious creation of the man and woman in Genesis 1–2 comes the tragic story of the fall in Genesis 3. The events chronicled therein do not tell a harmless story of the innocuous eating of a fruit God wanted to keep from Adam and Eve. It is a story of sin and rebellion perpetrated by God's image bearers, his vice-regents. Because of God's exalted status and the lofty position of the man and woman, the sin is treachery and betrayal at the highest levels. The result was cursing, death, and suffering. And it is all the fault of the first humans. Because of human sin, human suffering and human death entered the world.

Some suffering is the direct result of particular sins committed by the sufferer. Much suffering is the result of living in a broken and cursed world. But *all* suffering can be traced back to Genesis 3. The good news is that Jesus Christ came to save us from sin and lift the curse upon the cosmos, bringing an end to suffering, once and for all. The promise of the gospel is, "If you confess with your mouth, 'Jesus is Lord,' and believe in your heart that God raised him from the dead, you will be saved" (Rom. 10:9). Eternal suffering is not the destiny of the Christian.

The Bible's commitment to relief of suffering is demonstrated in the scriptural narratives and examples of Jesus and his apostles. For example, in response to the prayers of Hezekiah, the Lord determined to heal the king of Judah (2 Kings 20:5). Jesus' earthly ministry was characterized by healing those in need; he was troubled by human suffering and healed to relieve it (Matt. 14:14; 20:34; Mark 1:41; Luke 7:13). Jesus' healing ministry was a foretaste of the kingdom of God, evidence that the King of the kingdom was in the midst of the people (Matt. 12:22–28). The apostles healed as part of their kingdom proclamation (Acts 3:7; 5:16; 8:7; 9:34; 14:9–10; 28:8–9). Further, the New Testament elevates compassion and mercy as virtues that are to characterize God's people (Col. 3:12; James 3:17). Finally, Christians for millennia have been encouraged and inspired by the hope that one day all suffering will end. The apostle John wrote, "He will wipe away every tear from their eyes. Death will be no more; grief, crying, and pain will be no more, because the previous things have passed away" (Rev. 21:4).

So there is nothing sub-Christian about seeking relief from suffering, even by the ordinary means of doctors and medications. God cares deeply about the trials and pains of his people. For those who are suffering, the Lord is "the [God] who sees" (Gen. 16:13). He sees and collects all the tears of his saints (Ps. 56:8).

The ministry of Jesus Christ himself was characterized by healing those who were in

God cares deeply about the trials and pains of his people.

need (Matt. 4:23), so to end or reduce suffering is one of the paths of following Christ.

But the Scriptures also speak of the redemptive benefits of suffering. Even though suffering is the result of broken people living in a broken world full of other broken people, God uses suffering to bring about his good purposes in the life of every believer. Three passages will suffice to demonstrate this teaching.

James, the brother of Jesus, wrote, "Consider it a great joy, my brothers and sisters, whenever you experience various trials, because you know that the testing of your faith produces endurance. And let endurance have its full effect, so that you may be mature and complete, lacking nothing" (James 1:2–4). Here, James instructed Christians to rejoice in suffering because God uses trials to test the faith of the Christian. There is nothing distinct about the trials James commends. That is, followers of Christ ought not to think that the trial or suffering they are undergoing is not the kind James was talking about. While in *any* trial, Christians are to be confident that their loving God is using their suffering to test, prove, and strengthen their faith.

The first letter of the apostle Peter is full of encouragement to his readers to stay faithful in the face of persecution and suffering. One key to remaining steadfast is to see the hand of God in trials.

> You rejoice in this, even though now for a short time, if necessary, you suffer grief in various trials so that the proven character of your faith—more valuable than gold which, though perishable, is refined by fire—may result in praise, glory, and honor at the revelation of Jesus Christ. Though you have not seen him, you love him; though not seeing him now, you believe in him, and you rejoice with inexpressible and glorious joy, because you are receiving the goal of your faith, the salvation of your souls. (1 Pet. 1:6–9)

Like James, Peter instructed Christians to rejoice when suffering. Not because masochism is valued in Christian circles nor because Christians need to demonstrate how tough they are. No, Christians are to rejoice while suffering because God is at work in the heart of the suffering Christian, and the Lord who loves them will refine and purify their faith through the trial.

Finally, in 2 Corinthians 12, Paul records the strange affair of his thorn in the flesh:

> Therefore, so that I would not exalt myself, a thorn in the flesh was given to me, a messenger of Satan to torment me so that I would not exalt myself. Concerning this, I pleaded with the Lord three times that it would leave me. But he said to me, "My grace is sufficient for you, for my power is perfected in weakness."
>
> Therefore, I will most gladly boast all the more about my weaknesses, so that Christ's power may reside in me. So I take pleasure in weaknesses, insults, hardships, persecutions, and in difficulties, for the sake of Christ. For when I am weak, then I am strong. (2 Cor. 12:7–10)

We note that the suffering was caused by "a messenger of Satan," and was not the direct result of anything Paul had done. Paul desperately wanted relief and "pleaded with the Lord three times" that God would bring an end to the trial.

But God had goals beyond Paul's comfort. Paul learned to be humble, to depend on the Lord, and to trust in all circumstances. His attitude in the face of suffering was amazing and he remarkably was able to "take pleasure" in all his difficulties, not because he enjoyed them but because Christ's power was made manifest in the midst of them.

So relief of suffering is advocated in the Bible, but it is not the goal of the Christian faith to avoid suffering at any cost. While those saved by Christ need not fear eternal suffering, Jesus promised that trials and suffering would come to those who followed him (John 16:2–3). Paul warned the early Christians that they could not enter the kingdom apart from suffering (Acts 14:22), his goal was to know Christ and "the fellowship of his sufferings" (Phil. 3:10), and his own life was characterized by much hardship and trial (2 Cor. 11:24–33).

Our contemporary world, especially where I live in America, places a premium on pain avoidance. We don't like to suffer—not even a little—and it seems like there is no price we are unwilling to pay to escape the trials and traumas of this age. It is safe to say that relief of personal suffering is a higher priority to the world than it should be to the Christian.

Don't get me wrong. I am not saying Christians are called to suffer unnecessarily. When my head hurts, I pull out the Excedrin bottle. But is it possible, in our quest to quickly relieve suffering, that we are turning to mind-altering medication without proper reflection?

The Lord Often Uses Means to Heal

The Bible teaches that the Lord can heal miraculously. The Old and New Testaments abound with stories of God's intervening to heal without medicines or physical treatment (e.g., Gen. 20:17; 1 Kings 17:22; Matt. 4:24; Acts 3:1–10). When we are sick and suffering, we should absolutely pray for God to heal us, even miraculously.

As we consider biblical teaching that applies to medical marijuana, we must also observe that God often uses ordinary physical means to heal. For example, the Lord healed Hezekiah and saved his life through the application of a poultice of pressed figs (2 Kings 20:7). The Scriptures speak positively about bandages and medicine (e.g., Prov. 17:22; Ezek. 30:21; Luke 10:34). Luke was lauded for being a physician (Col. 4:14). Regardless of whether healing comes miraculously or through means explainable by science, the Lord is sovereign over our healing (Deut. 32:39). Therefore, the proper perspective of a Christian who has been healed through medicine or surgery is to thank the doctor *and* thank the Lord for healing through that doctor. Turning to medicine and depending on physician care are not acts of faithlessness. They are biblical and are ordinarily the means through which God will bring about healing. We should thank the Lord for good doctors and good medical treatments. He is sovereign over both.

Regardless of whether healing comes miraculously or through means explainable by science, the Lord is sovereign over our healing.

Is Pain Relief Justification for Other Side Effects?

Because medical marijuana and recreational marijuana are the same substance, the science is the same. So everything about how marijuana works covered in chapter 1 applies. Medical marijuana is a cannabinoid, and it activates the endocannabinoid receptors the same as recreational marijuana. The risks are the same also. Smoke from medical marijuana is dangerous to the lungs and heart. THC from medical marijuana intoxicates, and the Christian must consider if relief from suffering is worth the risks and problems with intoxication.

It is interesting that Jesus refused medication while on the cross. Mark 15:23 records that just prior to being crucified, "they tried to give him wine mixed with myrrh, but he did not take it." Why would Jesus do this? Jesus knew the cruelty of the cross. Just before his arrest, he was in such "anguish" that "his sweat became like drops of blood falling to the ground" as he prayed (Luke 22:44). The wine mixed with myrrh acted as a primitive narcotic that was charitably given to prepare the condemned for the crucifixion. But Jesus refused it. We are not told why.

Is it possible that Jesus wanted to face his work on the cross with a clear mind? The Scriptures nowhere prescribe this same approach to facing a difficult trial, but it is noteworthy that it was the path Jesus chose.

Is the Suffering Acute or Chronic?

Another consideration that weighs on the wisdom of the choice to take a mind-altering drug is the duration and intensity of the suffering. We commonly take anesthesia for surgery and are prescribed strong narcotics afterward for acute pain. No one should question the morality of that choice. These drugs are certainly mind-altering, but so is pain, especially acute pain. The world of the one suffering acute pain shrinks, and a clear perspective is difficult to maintain. The suffering can be so intense that thinking straight is impossible, judgment is impaired, and physical capacities are completely diminished. No one ought to find fault with people suffering from acute pain who choose to take a mind-altering drug for relief.

But is taking a psychoactive drug, such as an opioid or marijuana, the best way to treat chronic pain? To control chronic pain, one will have to regularly use the medication, which increases the likelihood of addiction if the medication is an opioid or marijuana (see chapter 2). Scripture is clear that addiction is wrong because it enslaves (2 Pet. 2:19). Remember that while marijuana is not as addictive as some substances, it is still addictive.

Opioids, however, are even more addictive than marijuana. If the prospect of addiction raises concerns about marijuana use for chronic pain, then those concerns ought to be multiplied for opioids. America is currently experiencing an opioid overdose and addiction epidemic. In 2012, a staggering 81.2 opioid prescriptions were dispensed for every one hundred people in America. That number is going down but was still at 51.4 prescriptions for every one hundred people in 2018.[1] Tragically, American opioid

---

[1] CDC, "U.S. Opioid Prescribing Rate Maps," Centers for Disease Control and Prevention, March 5, 2020, https://www.cdc .gov/drugoverdose/maps/rxrate-maps.html.

deaths spiked during the coronavirus pandemic that began in 2020.[2]

Many people who are now addicted to opioids, including some Christians, first took the drug as a prescription for relief of pain. What if those Christians who are now addicted to opioids had thought about the consequences of taking a highly addictive, mind-altering drug for chronic pain relief? Perhaps the questions Christians are asking today about the legitimacy of the medical use of marijuana have opened the space to consider the implications of taking other addictive mind-altering drugs. In other words, maybe the question of medical marijuana is prompting Christians to think biblically when it comes to prescribed drug use more generally.

Marijuana advocacy groups are hopeful that increased access to medical marijuana will lead to lower opioid addiction and mortalities. To this point the studies, while hopeful, have not been conclusive.[3] To be enslaved by an

---

[2] "Issue Brief: Reports of Increases in Opioid- and Other Drug-Related Overdose and Other Concerns during COVID Pandemic," October 6, 2020, https://www.ama-assn.org/system/files/2020-10/issue-brief-increases-in-opioid-related-overdose.pdf.

[3] John W. Finney, Keith Humphreys, and Alex H. S. Harris, "What Ecologic Analyses Cannot Tell Us About Medical Marijuana Legalization and Opioid Pain Medication Mortality," *JAMA*

opioid or marijuana is wrong and miserable. Before taking any mind-altering drug for a chronic condition, the Christian ought to consider the risks of addiction.

Because the Bible forbids intoxication, Christians ought to reflect on the wisdom of using marijuana, or any other mind-altering drug, to control pain. Remember, marijuana works as an intoxicant first and a pain reliever second, if at all.[4] Some theories speculate that there is no actual pain relief from marijuana; the marijuana instead serves to mellow the user so that he or she is not as bothered by the pain. But even if that is true, the chronic sufferer will often happily take even that kind of relief.[5] For most (not all) people, the amount of regular pot use necessary to curb chronic pain will be intoxicating. I covered the implications of taking an intoxicating substance for

---

Internal Medicine 175, no. 4 (April 1, 2015): 655–56, https://doi.org/10.1001/jamainternmed.2014.8006.

[4] Alison Mack and Janet Joy, *Marijuana as Medicine? The Science Beyond the Controversy* (Washington DC: National Academies Press, 2000), 81–82, https://www.ncbi.nlm.nih.gov/books/NBK224384/.

[5] For a helpful commentary on the decision to take edibles to manage severe pain, see Jeff Seidel, "I Swore I'd Never Touch Marijuana: Here's Why I Finally Did," *Detroit Free Press*, September 13, 2020, sec. Sports, https://www.freep.com/story/sports/columnists/jeff-seidel/2020/09/13/medicinal-marijuana-uses-nerve-pain/3472880001/.

the Christian in chapter 5. Those considerations do not completely disappear in the presence of pain and suffering. Peter's words still apply:

> Be sober-minded, be alert. Your adversary the devil is prowling around like a roaring lion, looking for anyone he can devour. Resist him, firm in the faith, knowing that the same kind of sufferings are being experienced by your fellow believers throughout the world. (1 Pet. 5:8–9)

Here Peter describes the Christian life as one that is to be lived in constant vigilance. Demonic forces seek to destroy, and Satan plays for keeps. The mind compromised by a psychoactive drug will be less able to resist the overtures of the enemy.

Before we move to pastoral concerns, let me state clearly that those who suffer acute and chronic pain have my deepest sympathies. My goal is not to condemn but to ask questions to aid in the quest for wisdom. There is no judgment intended on my part. Though I have not suffered personal pain either acutely or chronically, I have watched and walked with my wife who suffered extraordinarily through illness and treatment. I would have done anything in my power to alleviate the misery. I sympathize with the feelings of hopelessness and frustration that accompany suffering. I understand why someone would turn to medical marijuana in the hope that it might alleviate the suffering, if only just a little.

Pastoral Considerations and Questions

Here is a series of questions designed to help the pastor when approached by a congregant seeking counsel on whether to use marijuana for medical purposes. These questions can be easily modified for parents or anyone who is advising someone considering using medical marijuana.

Does the individual know all the implications?

During suffering, it is tempting to jump at anything that promises deliverance from the pain. But the Christian needs to know the medical risks and the problems a mind-altering drug like marijuana might pose to discipleship. When made aware of the risks or the impediments to discipleship, the price for relief might be judged to be too high. Walking through the risks covered in chapter 2 and the discipleship questions of chapter 5 will help the congregant make an informed decision about marijuana.

What malady will the medical marijuana treat?

In situations where a congregant comes to you requesting wisdom on whether to use medical marijuana, seek clarification on what is being treated. Is it a physician-diagnosed condition? If so, what are the treatment options? There may be other, better treatments available. Most people who have procured a medical marijuana card have done so for reasons other than a life-threatening illness. An overwhelming majority are given a medical marijuana card for pain maintenance.[6] Further, most card recipients do not fit the profile of the typical patient suffering from chronic pain, so a lot of people with medical marijuana cards are abusing the system.[7] A clear understanding of the malady or illness will enable you to give the best counsel.

---

[6] A 2014 study showed that almost 91 percent of medical marijuana users procured a medical marijuana card to alleviate acute or chronic pain. A small percentage cited a serious illness like AIDS or cancer. K. A. Sabet and E. Grossman, "Why Do People Use Medical Marijuana? The Medical Conditions of Users in Seven U.S. States," *Journal of Global Drug Policy and Practice* 8 (January 1, 2014): 1–26.

[7] Medical marijuana cardholders are disproportionately young and male while chronic pain patients are normally older and female. Ed Gogek, *Marijuana Debunked: A Handbook for Parents, Pundits and Politicians Who Want to Know the Case against Marijuana* (Ashville, NC: Chiron Publications, 2015), 112–14.

What is the extent of the suffering?

In addition to a clear diagnosis, inquiring about the level of suffering will also help you provide wise counsel. Because of the risk of addiction and the biblical prohibitions on intoxication, the decision to take a mind-altering drug should not be made lightly. In general, mind-altering drugs for acute pain taken in the short term do not present the same scope of problems that accompany mind-altering drugs for chronic pain taken over the long term.

Does the individual have a susceptibility to addiction or mental illness?

The statistics are clear that the odds of becoming addicted to marijuana increase the more regularly marijuana is used. Some people are more susceptible to substance addiction than others. The National Institute on Drug Abuse has provided a list of environmental risk factors to watch for, including a chaotic home and abuse environment, parents' use and attitudes toward drugs, peer influences, community attitudes, and low academic achievement. Biological risk factors that explain why some are more susceptible than others include genetics, gender, and the presence of mental disorders.[8] The more risk factors a person has, the greater the likelihood that drug use will lead to addiction.

What is the state of the individual's spiritual health?

People who are walking with the Lord are not immune to temptation, nor are they necessarily protected from the dangers associated with mind-altering drugs. But Christians who have wandered from the path of discipleship are already in a compromised position and are not in the best place to make decisions regarding medical drug use.

Can the individual take medical marijuana with a clear conscience?

The Scriptures are clear that whatever is not done in faith is sin (Rom. 14:23). If the individual cannot use marijuana with a clear conscience, then it will be sin, regardless of any other factors. Perhaps doubt will give way to persuasion at a later time, but until that time, the individual should abstain from marijuana and seek help from other sources.

---

[8] NIDA, "Drug Misuse and Addiction," National Institute on Drug Abuse, July 13, 2020, https://www.drugabuse.gov /publications/drugs-brains-behavior-science-addiction/drug-misuse -addiction.

Will medical marijuana use cause a problem for the individual's immediate family (children)?

Activities are never done in a vacuum. Children and other family members are always watching, and this is especially the case when a parent is suffering. The actions of the sufferer will give true testimony to the parent's convictions and faith. Will marijuana use compromise the child's resistance to future drug use? Will marijuana use create a home environment that is not conducive to bringing up children in the training and instruction of the Lord? Will secondhand smoke create a health hazard for the child? Will the user be able to parent responsibly while impaired? It is every parent's responsibility to ask such questions.

As you reflect on these questions, wrestling with whether or not to turn to marijuana in the hopes that it may offer some relief, remember that God is good. It is difficult to see clearly in the midst of suffering, but to the extent possible, focus on Jesus Christ and him crucified. If you want to know what God thinks of human suffering, of your suffering in particular, you need look no further than the cross. There, the love of God, comingled with his holiness, shouts his response to your trials. For there the Son of God died to take away your sin, to take away your shame, and to make possible the kingdom of God, when Jesus will usher in an eternal rule with no more trauma, no more suffering, and no more tears.

Questions and Answers for Pastors and Parents

This book is aimed toward Christians. Is it permissible for non-Christians to smoke pot?

There is only one God before whom all will stand, both Christians and non-Christians. There are not two different standards of morality by which people will be judged. Non-Christians, just like Christians, are created in the image of God and have been given a body in and for which they are to do the work of "imaging" or representing God.

What people do in their bodies matters to God, regardless of whether they are Christians. The health warnings apply to non-Christians just like Christians.

The major difference in the applicability of this book is that Christians, by definition, understand Jesus to be Lord. Much of the book does speak directly to disciples of Jesus, intentionally asking questions for which Christians properly ought to be concerned. I have no expectation that unbelievers want to honor Jesus in their thinking and actions. I do expect Christians to have those desires.

You gave some dire warnings concerning the health effects of marijuana. Why have I not heard these before?

I can think of three significant reasons that might be the case. First, because marijuana has been classified as a Schedule 1 drug, research has not been plentiful, and longitudinal studies have been difficult. So the limited amount of research contributes to the lack of public knowledge of the health risks.

Second, even when research is published, those seeking to disseminate it have to overcome a powerful and persuasive marijuana lobby. That lobby is well organized and well financed at both the political and media levels. We have seen just how efficient that lobby has been when we consider the speed at which legalization of recreational and medical marijuana has occurred at the state level. The marijuana lobby has been effective at promoting a narrative about marijuana and shutting down competing truth claims.[1]

Third, people have a strange devotion to marijuana and are relentless in their defense of the drug.[2] Rarely will anyone brag about their cocaine use. People usually do not even joke about drinking early in the morning. But marijuana advocates are often quick to trumpet their use and extol marijuana's benefits. "Wake and bake" is a humorous slang phrase that has made it into the urban vernacular, and if the aromas I encounter on my early morning runs through my Portland neighborhood are representative, it is a phrase that describes the marijuana use of a lot of people. Public devotion to marijuana does not create an environment where criticism of the drug is appreciated.

Is marijuana a gateway drug?

A gateway drug is understood to be a drug whose use can lead to the use of more dangerous drugs. With such a vague definition, it is difficult to identify "gateway

---

[1] Alex Berenson, *Tell Your Children: The Truth About Marijuana, Mental Illness, and Violence* (New York: Free Press, 2019), 229–39.

[2] Ed Gogek, *Marijuana Debunked: A Handbook for Parents, Pundits and Politicians Who Want to Know the Case against Marijuana* (Ashville, NC: Chiron Publications, 2015), 256–59.

drugs" with certainty. Studies have not been conclusive. Experience teaches that not all who use marijuana go on to harder drugs. But the National Institutes of Health does report that marijuana use "is likely to precede use of other licit and illicit substances," and cites medical research that posits biochemical reasons for why marijuana use will lead to other substance use disorders.[3] Additionally, addiction consultant and professor of psychiatry Dr. Kevin P. Hill has found in his research that "marijuana addiction can progress to addiction of other substances very quickly."[4]

Can I apply the arguments in this book to other drugs like mushrooms?

Yes. Absolutely.

The arguments presented against intoxication apply to any kind of mind-altering drug. Though this book is specifically about marijuana, I have tried to ask the kinds

---

[3] NIDA, "Is Marijuana a Gateway Drug?," National Institute on Drug Abuse, April 8, 2020, accessed September 25, 2021, https://www.drugabuse.gov/publications/research-reports/marijuana/marijuana-gateway-drug.

[4] Kevin P. Hill, *Marijuana: The Unbiased Truth About the World's Most Popular Weed* (Center City, MN: Hazelden Publishing, 2015), 25.

of questions a Christian can and should ask about any substance. The question of mushrooms might seem strange, but in my own home state, Oregonians, in the 2020 fall election, passed a ballot measure to create a program that would license providers to administer hallucinogenic mushrooms to people twenty-one years or older. (Did I mention that where I live is weird?)

What about microdosing THC for medical purposes?

Microdosing is the act of consuming a small amount of THC in order to reap some of the desired benefits without any of the negative effects (namely intoxication). Advocates argue that microdosing can be effective for such maladies as depression, chronic pain, anxiety, sleeplessness, and ADHD. Because not enough THC is consumed to create intoxicating effects, many of the concerns I raised about the mind-altering effects of medical marijuana do not apply. It is important to note that there is very little to no evidence that microdosing actually brings any of the proposed benefits. Further, I am concerned about the use of THC as a form of self-medication (in the same way that I would be concerned about someone who drank a glass of alcohol alone each night to help himself or herself relax). Though most people self-medicate with over-the-counter drugs (e.g., aspirin, cold medicine, etc.), my advice is to bring the "self-medication" into the open by speaking with a doctor for medical counsel or the elders of your church for the purposes of accountability and wisdom.

Isn't caffeine a mind-altering drug and addictive? How is caffeine any different from cannabis?

Caffeine is a mind-altering drug, a stimulant. But its psychoactive effects are not debilitating. Through its biochemical interaction with the human brain, it blocks sleep-inducing actions caused by natural chemicals and therefore speeds up nerve activity. The result is that it can temporarily make people feel alert and energetic. As such, it can be a useful tool and helpful for the various tasks to which we are called when we are not feeling alert and energetic.

Caffeine use contrasts favorably with marijuana, which typically leads to a weakened engagement, less clear thinking, and a distorted view of reality. But moderation with caffeine is a wise path to walk. Too much caffeine can cause sleeplessness, anxiety, digestive issues, and high blood pressure. People can develop a physical and even psychological dependence on the drug, and caffeine withdrawal will result in minor symptoms (compared to, say, opioid withdrawal) like headaches and irritability. But it is not addictive, at least not in the clinical sense. Caffeine use is not characterized by people making harmful decisions to self and others in order to make that next Starbucks run.

As a Christian parent, what should I do about my adult children who live with me and smoke pot?

If you live in a state where recreational marijuana is legal, this question is one of conscience and parental wisdom. It is never wise to violate one's conscience. If marijuana use violates your conscience, then you ought to forbid marijuana use in your home. It is appropriate to ask those living with you not to engage in behaviors you consider sinful or at least harmful. Parents have the right to establish the rules by which their adult children must abide if they are going to live in the parents' home.

The stakes are raised if there are underage children in the home. Influence on their behavior gives another reason to ask adult children to abstain. If your adult children cannot abide by the rules you have established for your house, it is appropriate to ask them to leave.

Should a church discipline over marijuana use? If so, when?

The basic steps of church discipline are outlined by Jesus in Matthew 18:15–20. They include (1) personal confrontation of the unrepentant sinner by a concerned or aggrieved party, (2) confrontation by two or more, (3) telling the church for the purpose of prayer and confrontation, and (4) removal of the unrepentant sinner from membership and fellowship in the church. The immediate context of Jesus' teaching in Matthew 18 indicates that the goals of church discipline always include the repentance, forgiveness, and restoration of the sinner (Matt. 18:1–14, 21–35).

Though we don't always think of it in these terms, anytime even the first step takes place, church discipline has occurred. The church should consider moving to the following steps when the sin is outward, serious, and unrepentant.[5] Unrepentant public intoxication through marijuana use would certainly meet those criteria. Before advancing to the third and fourth steps of church discipline (if not the second step), the elders of the church will need to be involved. Church leaders will have to consider whether the marijuana use is for medical purposes, the

---

[5] Jonathan Leeman, *Church Discipline: How the Church Protects the Name of Jesus* (Wheaton: Crossway, 2012), 74.

age of the user, whether responsibilities are being sinfully neglected due to marijuana use, and whether intoxication is occurring.

Are Christians morally obligated to vote against legalization in states that have not yet legalized marijuana?

As discussed in chapter 3, "The Christian and the Law," government has been ordained by God to promote the good and punish the bad for the purpose of human flourishing. But not everything the Bible defines as evil ought to be forbidden by law. Gluttony and pride were examples cited earlier of sinful behavior that government, in my opinion, ought not to prosecute. Therefore, I believe Christians of good will can disagree on whether government ought to forbid recreational or medical marijuana.

One Christian might be convinced that, because of the dangers listed in this book, the use of recreational marijuana ought to be forbidden by law. Another Christian might be equally convinced of the dangers but favor more limited government and would vote to legalize recreational marijuana. Another Christian might be concerned that criminalization of recreational marijuana has led to inequities in law enforcement, so would vote for legalization. The church ought to be careful not to bind the consciences of Christians on questions of wisdom and governmental policy.

How should a Christian interact with other believers who think differently on this issue?

Not all biblical truths and issues carry the same weight. I use the following categorization: some doctrines are worth *dying for* because to deny them would be to deny the gospel. Examples include the doctrines of the Trinity, the deity of Jesus Christ, and the inspiration of Scripture. Some doctrines are worth *dividing for*. That is, disagreement with another would not mean one was not a Christian, but it would make membership in the same church difficult. Examples include use of the sign gifts (tongues and prophecy) and whether to baptize infants. Some doctrines are worth *debating for*. You might passionately argue with a fellow church member, but you would do so in love, and it would not interfere with fellowship. Examples include the timing and nature of the millennium. And some doctrines are worth only *deciding for*. That is, they are not even worth debating. Examples include what happens to a person's clothes during the rapture.

The use of marijuana is not a "die for" issue. If church leaders are aware of a person's marijuana use and have not judged it to be sinful, then it is probably a "debate for" issue. You may well disagree with the leaders, but you do not have the right to carry out your own private church discipline on the marijuana user. If you are convinced in your own heart that the person's marijuana use is sinful and you cannot submit to your church's leaders, then it might be best for you to find a new church. Christians are obligated to show love and grace to one another (John 13:34–35). Disagreement over marijuana use among Christians who are not members of the same church should be an issue over which they agree to disagree.

What about vaping or edibles? Are they safer?

The American Lung Association has issued severe warnings against vaping (see chapter 2), so that does not seem like a safer option. Edibles present the advantage of entering the bloodstream through the digestion process, so the dangers to the lungs are not as great. Most users prefer smoking to edibles because the introduction of THC to the bloodstream is much quicker via the lungs than through the digestion process. One problem is that some inexperienced users end up ingesting too much marijuana through edibles because they do not feel themselves getting high and only feel the need to back off when it is too late. So, again, wisdom will need to be used, but I recommend rereading the more extensive comments on edibles above. While they are safer, it is still unwise for Christians to consume edibles.

I have heard that there is cannabis in the holy anointing oil of Exodus 30:23. Is it true that the Bible does not speak of marijuana?

Exodus 30:23 instructs that the making of the anointing oil is to include "fragrant cane" or "aromatic reeds." The Hebrew words are *qānŭ(h) bōsem*. Some marijuana advocates speculate that the *qānŭ(h) bōsem* refers to cannabis, implying that the holy anointing oil was psychoactive. There is no evidence that this is actually the case, and Hebrew scholars are happy with the translation "fragrant cane" or "aromatic cane." Recent archeological evidence has shown that cannabis and frankincense were found on an eighth-century BC "holy of holies" altar in Arad in Judea.[6] Faithful Israelite worship would have forbidden a temple in Arad, and that site is infamous for its syncretistic

---

[6] Taylor and Francis, "New Research Reveals Cannabis and Frankincense at the Judahite Shrine of Biblical Arad," Phys.org, May 29, 2020, https://phys.org/news/2020-05-reveals-cannabis-frankincense-judahite-shrine.html.

worship of Yahweh and Asherah. So it's not as though marijuana was unknown in ancient biblical times. But if it was used in worship, our only record right now is that it was used in blasphemous idolatry.